Before Dementia

20 questions
you need to ask
to help prevent
to prepare
to cope

Dr. Kate Gregorevic

Some of the names and identifying details of people mentioned in this book have been changed.

First published in English in Sydney, Australia, by HarperCollins Publishers Australia Pty Limited in 2023. This English language edition is published by arrangement with HarperCollins Publishers Australia PTY Limited.

Library of Congress Cataloging-in-Publication Data
is available through the Library of Congress

ISBN-13: 978-07573-2518-2 (Paperback)
ISBN-10: 07573-2518-1 (Paperback)
ISBN-13: 978-07573-2519-9 (ePub)
ISBN-10: 07573-2519-X (ePub)

Publisher: Health Communications, Inc.
        301 Crawford Boulevard, Suite 200
        Boca Raton, FL 33432-3762

Cover design by Mietta Yans, HarperCollins Design Studio
Cover image by istockphoto.com
Diagram on page 26 by istockphoto.com

Author photo by Rebecca Taylor

For the people living with dementia

and for those who love them

This book was written on the unceded lands of the Wurundjeri people. The land always was and always will be Aboriginal land.

Contents

Introduction

This is a book about dementia, and while there are elements of discovery and science, what it is really about is people. It's a book about living and of all the different things that happen to us from when we are born to when we get old. It's about the loss and grief that can accompany living with dementia. It's also about love and caring for others: the essence of humanity.

This book will have questions on biology and cells, questions on lifestyle and preventing dementia, and challenging questions about sex, death, and autonomy. It will explore why disease is a social construct—just as much as a biological construct—and what this means to living with or caring for someone with dementia.

In these pages I am going to ask you to engage with challenging ideas and topics that we don't discuss in everyday life. It is possible to spend most of our days avoiding difficult thoughts and conversations—it certainly feels comfortable to live this way—but if we don't engage with difficult issues, we are missing an essential part of what it means to be human. As humans we can imagine a future for ourselves; we can have empathy for others. This ability to think beyond our immediate circumstances and connect is the best thing about us.

In writing this book, I also had to ask *myself* difficult questions. People with very advanced dementia, who have lost language ability, cannot consent to be part of a book to help understand the disease. Many can't speak in their own words about their experience. One of the reasons I wrote this book is to reduce stigma around dementia. I want people to recognize that even in its late stages, people living with dementia are still people trying to make sense of the world and to seek connection. Yet, I did not want to breach the privacy of my patients, so unless I had explicit permission from someone who could give consent, the stories shared with you are constructs to best demonstrate the breadth of human experience that I have encountered in the course of my work.

In my clinical work, I see many patients with advanced dementia. Some of these people are content, but many are distressed. I also speak to many caregivers who experience complex feelings. They love the person with dementia, they want to give them the best care possible, but they are also enduring grief and sometimes burnout. I don't want to worsen the fear of dementia, but I also want to respect the gamut of feelings of people who have shared their situations with me. Acknowledging the broad experience is part of improving care for people with dementia and supporting those who love and care for them.

This book might be uncomfortable reading at times, because it is uncomfortable to sit with ambiguity and uncertainty and to explore difficult topics and preconceived ideas, but I hope that in reading it, you will come away with an increased ability to understand some of the most complex aspects of being human. Facing our own mortality and uncertain future is unsettling, but if we don't do this, we miss the full richness of what it is to be alive.

A person living with dementia is not defined by their illness, but their illness is still a large part of their life. Part of breaking down stigma is considering the language we use. Using disrespectful language causes harm and can diminish the personhood of someone living with dementia. To that end, I have used the phrases "person with dementia" and "person living with dementia." Language can be tricky to always get right, but the key guiding principle is to be respectful. The Dementia Australia language guidelines state, "It is important to use language that focuses on the abilities (not deficits) of people living with dementia to help people stay positively and meaningfully engaged, and retain feelings of self-worth."

On a personal note, writing this book was an emotional process for me because I didn't realize how much work I needed to do in breaking down my own fears around dementia. It was also incredibly rewarding. The science of how our brains work, as well as what can go wrong, is deeply fascinating, especially in the context of the social and economic factors that influence biology. I spent time thinking about the broader issues of health and caring and have strengthened my resolve to end the stigma.

Most importantly, writing this book has improved my understanding and connection with the people I meet who are living with dementia. I hope that you find reading it just as interesting and rewarding.

Dr. Kate Gregorevic

What is dementia and are you at risk?

It's the end of my first consultation with Dulcie and her daughter Barbara. Dulcie has had dementia for many years. Barbara is struggling because Dulcie has been getting up multiple times a night, thinking it is morning and trying to go outside. Barbara wants to continue caring for her mother at home, but she is exhausted. She wants to know how to get help.

At the end of the appointment, I ask Barbara and Dulcie if they have any final questions. Barbara pauses a moment and then asks, a little embarrassed, "What is dementia?"

Barbara was embarrassed to ask this question because she felt like she should already know the answer. One of the best things about little kids is they have no qualms about admitting a gap in their knowledge. For some reason, part of reaching adulthood is becoming self-conscious about not knowing something, a barrier that overrides curiosity. The problem with going through life embarrassed to admit to a gap in our knowledge is that it means missing opportunities to learn.

Barbara is a caregiver and lived-experience expert, and so she understands that the question "What is dementia?" is actually very hard to answer.

Dementia occurs when a disease or progressive processes cause damage, and brain function is impaired enough to impact everyday life. The symptoms of dementia are the result of a brain that is no longer able to correctly take in information, interpret it, and act on it. Dementia is a "syndrome," or a collection of symptoms, and it can be caused by many different diseases. The onset of dementia is generally slow and gets worse over time. While there are common symptoms of dementia, it is nevertheless unique and individual to every person, because our social roles differ by age, gender, education, household, family structure, and geography.

The word "dementia" is an umbrella term for multiple diseases that cause damage to the cells of the brain, stopping them from being able to function and so leading to progressive decline in memory and thinking. These diseases often have overlap in symptoms, risk factors, and in the challenging questions they raise about autonomy and care. Unless otherwise specified, when I use the word "dementia," I am talking about *all* the diseases that cause dementia.

It is also important to distinguish dementia from the disease process that is causing the damage in the brain. The damage in the brain can start decades before any symptoms of dementia. This means there isn't a clear day when someone goes from cognitively intact to having a cognitive disability. It's also important to keep in mind that not everyone with damage to the brain will have the same symptoms or indeed any symptoms at all.

Dementia is in the category of neurodegenerative disorders—where there is progressive damage to the brain and nervous system by a disease process—and, usually many years after diagnosis, it is fatal.

The early symptoms of dementia are subtle and insidious, but the final stages, when someone loses words, and the ability to walk, chew, and swallow, are stark and terrifying. Dementia is the leading cause of death for women in Australia. As I mentioned in my introduction, I have seen the final stages of dementia up close many times, when people lose most of their words and can't recognize their loved ones. It is heartbreaking for families and unsettling to think that could be my fate one day.

Barbara's question about what dementia actually is was not at all foolish or something to be embarrassed about. Rather, it was the first step toward a difficult but necessary conversation. In our society, unless you do a job like mine, it is very easy to avoid thinking about death. We have a medical system that is set up for cure and intervention rather than caring. Unless you have spent time with people with advanced dementia, and sat with some difficult thoughts, the choices in the final stages of the disease can come as a shock.

How common is dementia?

You probably know—or knew—someone with dementia. Enough of us do to suggest that the condition is common, but the question of *how* common is very difficult to answer.

The Australian Institute of Health and Welfare estimates that there are around 400,000 people in Australia—out of a population of nearly 26 million people—living with dementia and that two-thirds are women. This is an estimate, and part of the reason is because there are a lot of people who have undiagnosed dementia. I know because I meet them when they come to the hospital for another reason, and their cognitive deficits become obvious in the stressful and unfamiliar environment they find themselves in, away from their family.

Part of getting an accurate population estimate depends on considering cultural, social, and educational factors. Although the Australian Institute of Health and Welfare has estimated that two-thirds of people with dementia are women, the question of whether women are at a higher risk of dementia than men is difficult to answer, and depends on many variables, particularly considering women have a longer average life expectancy.

The Chicago Health and Aging study ran from 1993 to 2011 with in-person interviews of over 10,000 individuals every three years. For a subset of 842 people, the study also included a battery of cognitive tests. In this cohort, women and men were at equal risk of developing dementia. Another cohort involved in the Rush Memory and Aging Project, which had 785 participants who did not have dementia at baseline, showed no difference between men and women.

Interestingly it may be that geography has something to do with it. Studies in Europe and Asia have found that dementia is more common in women, whereas studies in the United States, such as those previously mentioned, have shown that this is not the case. As you will learn later, tests of memory are influenced by education, and many women in these older sample groups would have had less education than men, something many studies did not measure.

Nevertheless, one reason that women might seem to be at higher risk of dementia is because of their longer life expectancy. Since more women live into very old age, and this is the time when dementia risk is highest, longevity certainly accounts for some of that two-thirds number. Women also tend to survive longer after a dementia diagnosis, and surviving with a condition means you can be counted in a prevalence study.

Would you want to know if you are at risk of dementia?

The only place Nicole feels like she can speak openly is in her Facebook group for other young people who are caregivers for people with dementia. At university, the other students are worried about what their plans are for Saturday, who kissed whom, or planning a wild backpacking trip around South America. Nicole can't stand those conversations. Instead, she comes straight home after class, her body tense until she gets inside and finds that her mother is still in the house and hasn't gone for a walk and become lost again. Nicole makes sure her sisters have dinner and do their homework, then she cleans and folds washing. She checks the bank balance to make sure her mother's disability pension will stretch for the week.

At the end of the day, Nicole is usually too busy to stop and think about whether she is also going to get dementia.

Younger onset dementia is rare, yet it can happen. The most common genes that carry the mutation are the gene for the amyloid precursor protein, and genes called "presenilin1" and "presenilin2." These genetic mutations are autosomal dominant with complete penetrance. In other words, if you carry one copy of the gene, you are guaranteed to get younger onset dementia, most commonly in your forties, after you have already had your own children.

For people with younger onset dementia, and their children, a simple blood test will show whether they have these genes. Getting a blood test is easy; the difficult part is deciding whether you want to live your life always wondering if today is the day symptoms will start to appear. The rare families who carry this genetic mutation will have seen other people they love develop younger onset dementia; they will possibly have experienced being a caregiver.

While there are some rare familial cases of dementia, in which people inherit a gene that guarantees they will get dementia, usually in their forties or fifties, this accounts for less than 1 percent of cases. Dementia is usually a polygenic disease, meaning that there are multiple genes that can add or take away a little bit of risk, all while interacting with lifestyle factors. Testing for single gene mutations, like the ones mentioned above, is only available after genetic counseling, because this information has serious psychological implications.

The most common gene that increases the risk of dementia generally, as opposed to younger onset dementia, is apolipoprotein E allele 4 (APOEe4). The APOE gene makes a protein that carries cholesterol around in the blood. There are different forms or "alleles" of this gene: APOEe2, APOEe3, and APOEe4. Around 10 to 15 percent of the population will have Alzheimer's disease by the age of eighty-five. If you have one copy of APOEe4, the risk is 25 to 40 percent, and for those with two copies of the gene the risk is 40 to 55 percent. Finding out you have one or two copies of the APOEe4 allele doesn't mean you are certain to get Alzheimer's disease, but it does mean having to settle in with the knowledge that it is a distinct possibility.

While it is possible to get this test after seeing your doctor, there are now a plethora of companies that will analyze your genes for a fee. All you need to do is swab the side of a cheek, post your swab off, and you can get a report that tells you whether or not you carry the APOEe4 allele.

We have a saying in medicine that you shouldn't do a test unless the answer will change your management. While there are potential benefits of finding out that you have the APOEe4 gene, such as increased motivation to incorporate positive health behaviors into your lifestyle, there are also harms, like emotional distress. I would certainly advise taking time to think carefully whether you really want to know this information, particularly as there is no current medical therapy to decrease the risk.

Also, this gene test doesn't help us diagnose dementia. If someone has a clinical history that is consistent with dementia, knowing their genetic status won't help me or other doctors work out whether the person has dementia or not, as plenty of people still have dementia without carrying a high risk gene and vice versa.

Many people report that in the long term they are happy to know they are at risk because they have made positive lifestyle changes, such as getting more exercise, sleeping better, and improving cardiovascular risk factors for conditions, including diabetes and hypertension. I would argue these are things we should all be doing anyway.

Personally, I do not want to know whether or not I have the APOEe4 allele. It won't change my behavior because I already prioritize healthy behaviors. As a doctor, I am extremely familiar with the many different accidents and diseases that can befall someone, and while I am very invested in prevention, I am also pragmatically aware that there are no guarantees.

I know that some people will feel differently. I would always suggest that people speak with their own doctor, and ideally a genetic counselor, before sending off a test in the mail. There is also the online decision tool: gene test or not (genetestornot.org), which can help you think through the issues before you make a decision.

Test before symptoms

One important distinction is that between a screening test and a diagnostic test. A screening test is something that is done when someone has no symptoms. For example, when you turn fifty in Australia, you receive a bowel cancer screening kit in the mail. The basic idea here is that you can send in a tiny sample of your stool to a lab to look for blood. If this test returns positive, you will go on to have a colonoscopy, which is a diagnostic test. If the colonoscopy shows bowel cancer in an early stage, it can be removed during the colonoscopy. If someone notices that they have blood in their stool, they don't need a screening test; they need investigations to diagnose the cause of their symptoms. As I have mentioned, diagnosing dementia is a clinical process. But what about screening for dementia?

In 2020, the US Preventive Services Task Force reviewed the evidence on screening for dementia and concluded that it was insufficient to make a recommendation because there was not enough evidence to evaluate the harms and benefits of such an act. Neither was there enough evidence to evaluate the harms and benefits of a screening test, like asking a series of questions to test cognitive abilities. This might seem strange, because what harm could there be in giving someone a disease label? In fact, giving someone the label of a terminal neurological disease has serious implications, and many people might experience significant distress as a consequence.

Others argue there are advantages to identifying cognitive decline before it impacts day-to-day life because it can help people plan for their future or access support or formal services. Another advantage of screening is that it might pick up a decline in cognition due to a treatable cause, like depression, insomnia, or medication, although in this case the person being screened is not strictly asymptomatic as they have insomnia or depression. Early cognitive decline identified on a screening test might give the opportunity to go into a clinical trial to further progress the science and test a potential benefit along the way.

It's important to keep in mind that a screening test is not the same as a diagnostic test. Screening tests are supposed to identify which people need further investigation to rule in or out a diagnosis. Screening tests are designed to be quick and easy. In screening, we talk about sensitivity and specificity. "Sensitivity" means a test shouldn't have too many false negatives; "specificity" means a test shouldn't have too many false positives. If the pass mark for a screening test for dementia was set at passing a university math exam, most of us would fail and therefore be flagged as a false positive of being at risk for dementia. Conversely, if the screening test was being able to remember our name and birthdate, almost everyone would pass.

To complicate this even further, the screening tests we have—like the Mini-Mental State Examination (MMSE), a test of various domains of cognitive function that is scored out of 30 and takes 5 to 10 minutes to complete—are heavily influenced by factors such as education. Let's say we use a cutoff tally of 25 correct answers out of 30 as a grade for the marker for when people should have further assessments for dementia.

Consider my first patient, a man who started his own highly successful business, which is now run by his daughter. He scores 28 out of 30. My second patient is a woman who was born overseas, has English as a second language, and is not literate. She scores 21 out of 30.

Then consider the wider context of these two examples. The businessman, Claude, lives with his wife and goes to the office every day, but he is no longer doing any actual work. His family is very aware that his memory is a problem and have put in many compensatory strategies. Despite his high score, and after further testing and clarifying interviews with his family, it is determined that he does have dementia.

Eudoxia, who scored 21 out of 30, was in the hospital with a broken arm, so she couldn't do the drawing components of the test, and English is not her first language. However, she is able to listen and learn from the occupational therapist to develop strategies to compensate for her broken arm, and she is able to talk through the ways she plans to sort out tasks like dressing herself and preparing food. She can remember and problem solve. It is clear she does not have dementia.

One of the reasons we don't have evidence for the risks and benefits of dementia screening is simply because the tests we use aren't great for a large subset of the population. Screening people with no or even mild symptoms also has another risk: overdiagnosis.

What is overdiagnosis?

A few years ago, I somehow got a scratched cornea in the middle of the night. I didn't end up sleeping much due to the excruciating pain. The next day, I went to work and I could not remember what was wrong with any of my patients. Embarrassingly, I also forgot the name of a colleague I knew well.

I didn't go and get any follow-up memory tests. Instead I got a bit more sleep and everything went back to normal. Certain brain functions, like memory and problem-solving, are highly sensitive to things like sleep deprivation or stress.

It seems simple and straightforward that someone with memory problems should get assessed to see if they would be given a diagnosis of dementia, but there is such a thing as *overdiagnosis*.

One group of patients I look after is people older than sixty-five admitted through the trauma unit. When people come in with trauma they have what we call a "pan-scan." Basically, they get a CT scan that goes from their head to their hips to look for any unrecognized injuries. In people ages sixty-five and older, this will almost always show up "incidentalomas." "Incidentalomas" is a quasi-medical term that refers to abnormalities we see on scans done for other reasons. We find these because, with so many people being scanned, there will almost always be a part of the body that looks a little different from what we expect. We are often then obliged to follow these up with further investigations, such as colonoscopies or additional CTs, to look at the injury in more detail. Sometimes, this is valuable. We might find an otherwise healthy seventy-year-old with an early bowel cancer (although hopefully this wouldn't happen because this seventy-year-old should be participating in a bowel cancer screening program), and so on.

When we find incidentalomas in someone who is ninety-five, it's a different story. People who are ninety-five are invariably frail, so any medical procedure, even a minor one like a colonoscopy, needs to be considered very carefully because it can cause more harm than good. Even if my ninety-five-year-old patient does have a cancer in their bowel, they may not have the physiological reserve to make a good recovery from a curative surgery. There is also an excellent chance they will die of something else before the bowel cancer ever causes a symptom. That initial pan-scan can start a trajectory of investigations and treatment that does nothing to help someone achieve a longer and better quality of life.

Overdiagnosis is an increasingly recognized problem in medicine. We screen for all sorts of conditions, such as diabetes, prediabetes, high blood pressure, breast cancer, prostate cancer, and high cholesterol. The entire point of screening and early diagnosis is to treat early enough to make a difference to quality of life. It assumes disease follows a straight line and will always progress in a straightforward fashion. Therefore, preventative strategies and early intervention are incredibly important. A good example of this is treating high blood pressure in midlife, which protects the health of brain blood vessels. For other conditions testing isn't so straightforward. Prediabetes, for example, means having slightly elevated blood sugars. In a study of adults of an average age of seventy-five with prediabetes it was shown that it was actually more common for them to return to normal blood sugar levels than to progress to diabetes. In these cases, the label of "prediabetes" did nothing to improve health outcomes.

For someone who is younger and has memory problems, especially if the problems are impacting their paid and unpaid work, it is very important to undergo a full evaluation for dementia. For someone who is frail with a limited life expectancy, the benefits are far less clear. Once we arrive at a label, what does it change?

Mild cognitive impairment (MCI) is considered a precursor state to dementia: a step along the road. The problem is that most people "diagnosed" with mild cognitive impairment will not progress to dementia. Often studies that look at the rates of conversion from MCI to dementia recruit patients who have been seen at a memory clinic. This means that they, or someone who knows them well, was worried enough to seek a specialist medical opinion to get the diagnosis. This means that there is already a noticeable problem, as these people are different from a group of truly asymptomatic people. In one particular research study, reseachers compared people who had been diagnosed with MCI because they went to a clinic with others who had been identified through screening. After around two to three years, 13 percent of the people who had sought help at a specialized memory clinic and been diagnosed with mild cognitive impairment had progressed to dementia, compared with 3 percent of people who were diagnosed after the asymptomatic screening. This highlights a fundamental problem with estimating how many people will convert from MCI to dementia in a year: many studies rely on people who have decided to get help because they are worried about their memory, compared to someone who has no concerns in everyday life.

What we can draw from the previous study is that if people already had functional impairment, by definition, their cognitive decline was already significant. Since the majority of people with mild cognitive impairment won't progress to dementia, it is not a meaningful label. Screening asymptomatic people in the community, putting them through further cognitive assessment, then giving this label is an example of overdiagnosis, because it absolutely does not mean there will be progression.

To screen or not to screen?

Medical testing for the sake of medical testing is not a good thing. The young woman with the 50 perfect chance of carrying a gene that guarantees dementia might want to know this before she decides to start a family. It might influence the choices she makes through life. It might also be a heartbreaking burden for her to know that she is destined to get the same disease that she might have nursed a beloved parent through. A diagnosis might also lead to nights lying awake, worrying about future memory loss.

Knowing you carry the APOEe4 gene might inspire a healthier lifestyle, although I would argue that if we care about brain health we should all be doing this anyway.

Since we don't have a treatment that will alter the course of dementia (which I discuss later), the other question is whether screening will improve quality of life. To me, it's hard to see how this can be the case. The entire premise of screening is that it is a test being done before symptoms. If there are no symptoms and the cognitive deficits are not impacting quality of life, then quality of life is hard to improve.

For someone with no symptoms, a poor performance on a screening test could lead them down a long diagnostic pathway to get a label that won't impact treatment or everyday life. As I have said, this is especially true for someone who is older, living with frailty and multiple medical problems, and who has a limited life expectancy.

Conversely, a screening test in someone highly educated *with* symptoms may offer false reassurance. A wife who has brought her highly educated husband to see the GP for his memory problems and personality change, who is told that he is fine because he got a high score on the screening test, will still be left with the problem of a husband with a failing memory and personality change who needs a more detailed workup.

Let's also pretend that we have a medication that will stop dementia, but it has a 10 percent risk each year of severe side effects such as brain swelling and small bleeds. For the woman with a gene mutation that guarantees dementia, this may be worth trying. For someone with the APOEe4 gene, this decision is not quite as straightforward. They are far from guaranteed to get dementia, so starting a medication that they would need for decades, with serious potential side effects, carries significant risk. Even for someone with mild cognitive impairment that is not actually impacting day-to-day life, and who is very unlikely to progress to dementia, such a drug is likely to be too risky to consider.

Currently, dementia screening, by doing tests before someone has symptoms, is not recommended. This may change one day in the future. Swabbing your cheek and sending it away for an anonymous analysis to get back a report with cold, hard numbers is easy. Knowing what to do with that information is not.

The reality is that no matter your genetic profile, just by living and getting older, you have a risk of dementia because we are not in perfect control of our health. One of the fundamental challenges of life with a human brain so capable of imagination is sitting with that uncertainty and choosing to live as well as possible anyway.

What are the symptoms of dementia?

Rose

When it was sheepshearing time, it was all hands on deck. At around 10 a.m., Bruce would stick his head in to tell Rose how many to expect for lunch. Whether it was ten, twenty, or even forty, everyone always knew they were in for a great feed with Rose. Even if there were a few more than she planned for, she could stretch the stew with extra potatoes or bake another loaf of bread, and the men always went back to their work talking about what a great cook the missus was.

Bruce and Rose were a team. He worked the fields, managed the sheep, and kept the fences repaired while she kept the garden and the house, got the kids to and from school, did the laundry, and, of course, did the cooking. No one had ever seen a prouder husband the year Rose won the prize for the best sponge cake at the local show.

When Bruce died, Rose couldn't bear to stay on the farm. It was time for their oldest son to take over, so she went to live in town near her daughter, Sue. Everyone helped Rose with the cleaning and the cooking, and when Sue's husband remarked that he couldn't remember the last time Rose had made a sponge, Sue thought her mom was probably just tired. She was pretty old, after all.

Sue dropped by most days, bringing meals and doing the laundry. Her mom's memory was going a bit, but she was sure it was just age. The day Sue went to visit and found a terrible smell of burnt plastic and the kettle on the stove, she became anxious. A few weeks later, when Rose asked when Bruce would be home, Sue had to go to the front of the house and cry. Then she made an appointment to see the doctor.

After the doctor confirmed Rose had dementia, Sue thought for a long time about when it all started. Was it when her mom stopped making the sponge cakes? Looking back, Sue realized things hadn't been right for a while, but no matter how she tied herself in knots, she couldn't quite pin it down.

When you can't look away

The onset of dementia is so insidious that it often takes something really obvious, an example of memory loss that is so stark, so unforgiving, that it is impossible to look away. This is often when the reframing begins, when all the little things that were so small in themselves start to coalesce. At the time, no one noticed when Rose stopped baking cakes, but Sue now realizes it was because Rose couldn't remember how.

Symptoms are very important to doctors when we are making a diagnosis. They are usually defined as a physical or mental problem a patient experiences. A symptom is something that is experienced, like an itch, rather than a sign someone can see, like a rash.

People experiencing symptoms of dementia can't always describe them, nor are they always apparent to the person experiencing them. In the story above, Rose does not remember that Bruce is dead, so she is not aware there is a problem. A sign like a rash is clear and visible, measurable, and objectively present to the person with the rash and anyone looking at it; a symptom is something that is experienced by the individual and may be more or less noticeable to those around them.

For some people the symptoms of dementia will cause problems quickly, particularly if the person is young and still working. For others, for example, if they are not working and have a family to cocoon them, their cognitive decline may go unnoticed for a long time in the supportive embrace of their family's care.

How does a brain work?

To understand the symptoms of dementia, it is worth taking a small detour to understand exactly how a brain works. The primary purpose of a brain is to sense and interpret the environment, so we can move around to fulfill our needs (such as securing food or safety). Even the simplest animals have a brain—a small collection of nerve cells to process sensory information—but no animal has a brain as capable of complex thought as humans do. Nor does any animal have a brain as big for its body size as the human brain. One of the reasons animals ration their brain size is that brains are energetically ravenous organs. In humans they make up around 2 percent of our body weight but use 20 percent of our energy.

Every cell in our body carries the same genetic information but, depending on what their job is, they can look very different. The cells of the brain are highly specialized for their important functions. Our brains have billions of nerve cells, or neurons, which form branching communication networks. These neurons have a "head" with lots of sites for connection, and a tail that can, in turn, connect with other cells. We have around a thousand trillion connections in our brain. I'm not even going to pretend I can conceptualize that number!

Electrical impulses travel along the nerve cells and, when they get to the end, cause the release of a chemical substance called a "neurotransmitter." Depending on the neurotransmitter, this can make the next cell along either more or less active.

It is these connections between cells that allow a brain to function. When we are babies, our brain cells are busy making connections with one another, called synapses. The number of these actually peaks at age three. These are then "pruned" down to the most used pathways. These pathways are not fixed over life, which is why we continue to learn, a concept called brain plasticity. While the developing brain of a child has more plasticity than an adult, this is not completely lost over life.

The brain also has other cells that support the neurons. These are called "glial" cells. The word "glia" comes from "glue." Scientists initially thought they were the glue that holds the neurons together, but now we know they have a critical role in brain function. There are three different types of glia cells. *Microglia* are the immune cells of the brain. They scan for damage and foreign invaders. Microglia also have an important role in pruning synapses between cells in development, as well as maintaining them in a healthy brain. *Astrocytes* contribute to keeping the environment just right for the neurons by making sure they are relatively protected from fluctuations in the rest of the body. *Oligodendrocytes* make myelin, which coats the nerve cells to allow electrical messages to travel through them faster.

All these support cells are critical for our brains to function properly, which means being able to understand and act on what we sense, as well as plan for the future.

How do we think?

It fills me with wonder every time I try to conceptualize how a group of cells, with electrical signals and chemicals, translate to the glorious abilities of human existence, including answering something as banal as the question: "What did you have for breakfast today?"

Different parts of the brain have different functions. As an example, the *frontal lobes* control movement and speech, and help us control emotions rather than act out the first thing that pops into our heads. The *parietal lobes* are involved in interpreting touch, such as when you hold a coin in your hand and know what it is, as well as understanding where our bodies are located in space. The *occipital lobes* at the back of the brain interpret the light signals that come in through the eyes.

FUNCTIONAL AREAS OF THE BRAIN

LATERAL VIEW

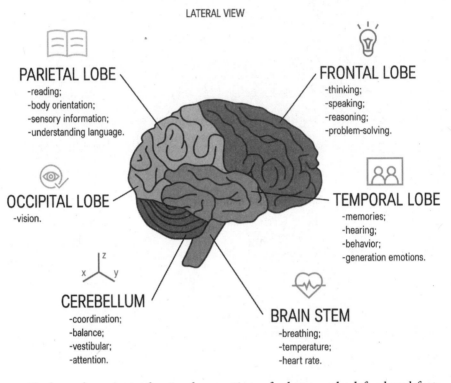

PARIETAL LOBE
-reading;
-body orientation;
-sensory information;
-understanding language.

FRONTAL LOBE
-thinking;
-speaking;
-reasoning;
-problem-solving.

OCCIPITAL LOBE
-vision.

TEMPORAL LOBE
-memories;
-hearing;
-behavior;
-generation emotions.

CEREBELLUM
-coordination;
-balance;
-vestibular;
-attention.

BRAIN STEM
-breathing;
-temperature;
-heart rate.

Back to the seemingly simple question of what you had for breakfast: Let's consider what's involved. First, the sound waves enter through your ears, then cells in the inner ear convert these to electrical signals that travel back to the auditory cortex in the temporal lobe, where an important part of the brain called Wernicke's area helps decode the words. If this part of the brain does not work, you cannot understand language, and while people produce speech, the words make no sense. The temporal lobe also contains key memory structures, which are needed to recall the information about your meal; the memory is turned into words in Broca's area in the frontal lobe, which is right next to the motor cortex of the brain (also in the frontal lobe); this causes the muscles of the larynx and mouth to form words to answer the question. Nearly the whole brain is involved in responding to the question.

We can add another layer of complexity. Let's say your breakfast was awful and the person who cooked it asks eagerly if you liked it. Your frontal lobe would consider the other person's feelings and weigh up giving an honest answer: Will you answer honestly to ensure that you never need to eat that awful meal again or will you resort to lying to protect their feelings?

These simple, everyday interactions show just how complex and integrated our brain function is: if any of the parts of the brain that control a function are damaged, or the connections between are damaged, it won't be possible to answer this question.

The damage predicts the disability

Since dementia usually occurs in older adults, it is rarely framed in terms of disability, but disability is a result of the cognitive decline. By the time someone has symptoms of dementia, cells and structures within the brain are damaged. One of the reasons the symptoms of dementia can vary is that the damage can be in different parts of the brain. Even Alzheimer's disease, characterized by the buildup of abnormal proteins, won't always have the same symptoms. While most people develop memory loss early, someone could have other uncommon early symptoms, such as an inability to interpret visual information, because their damage is in the back of the brain.

While some of the different diseases that cause dementia will have specific symptoms, such as the personality change that comes with frontotemporal dementia, this is not always clear-cut. It is just one of the challenges in working out which type of dementia a person has, and what is actually going on in the cells of the brain to cause the damage in the first place.

What are the symptoms of dementia?

A common misunderstanding about dementia is that it is just memory loss. While this is a common early symptom, there are many other symptoms, depending on which part of the brain is damaged. Dementia usually progresses slowly; if someone has a sudden change in their memory and thinking, this is likely to be caused by something different.

Memory

As you will learn over the coming pages, memory depends on a complex integration of many parts of the brain. Since it is so complex it is also very sensitive, which makes it vulnerable when there is damage in the brain. The memory loss that most people associate with dementia is short-term memory loss, that is, rapidly forgetting new information and having trouble learning new things. As the disease progresses, older memories are affected. This can extend to forgetting procedural skills, like how to get dressed.

Why is memory so often a problem in dementia?

While certain brain structures, such as the hippocampus, are key for memory, actual memories are more like a collection of mental abilities that depend on different systems within the brain. A memory system is a way of processing and storing information that will be used at a later time.

Memory is created by neurons (nerve cells) communicating in a pattern. In a fascinating study, researchers implanted electrodes in the brains of rats to measure which parts of the brain were active while they learned to navigate a maze. They then looked at the rats during sleep and found that the exact same neurons were firing, but faster. What they concluded was that during the dream phase of sleep, the rats were consolidating the memory of the maze. (This is why our bodies are paralyzed when we dream, so we don't try to physically act them out!)

Memory can be explicit (what's your address?) or implicit (knowing how to ride a bike). There are different systems for different types of memories. Semantic memory refers to things we know, like stating a fact. Episodic memory is remembering things in a personal context, such as what you did on your last birthday. Procedural memory is remembering how to do things, such as tie your shoelaces or drive or ride a bike, which you would be aware are memories that last over time. Working memory is information we need only for a short time, usually to do a specific task. Working memory means you are able to manipulate information in your mind (what's seventy-three plus fifty-five?), and it stays in your mind for seconds to minutes.

Researchers have learned a lot about the brain by studying neuroimaging and people with diseases or injuries that impact particular brain structures, and this relates to memory as well. For example, procedural memory involves the movement parts of the brain, and episodic memory involves the temporal lobes. This is why disease processes that impact different parts of the brain can cause different types of memory dysfunction. If, for example, there is damage to the frontal lobes, which function like a computer to bring out memories in the right context, there can be a disconnect with reality and false memories can be recalled. An extreme case of this is "confabulation," which occurred in a patient I saw who had spent weeks in the hospital but who told me a coherent story about going on a plane to a beach holiday the day before.

There are a few unusual people who have the capacity to remember everything they have done throughout their lives. Most of us are not like this. Memories from long ago fade out over time. However, memories associated with strong emotion can be more persistent, and this is due to the impact of stress hormones on the brain. From an evolutionary perspective, this is helpful: you don't go back to the spot where you were nearly eaten by a lion. But it can also have negative effects, as seen in post-traumatic stress disorder when people get vivid flashbacks and nightmares triggered by recalling an event or experiencing something similar.

Often, the memories that are most solid are our oldest. Perhaps because these are the ones we have had a chance to run through the most times. People with dementia will often go back to an earlier time in their life, and we need to meet them there.

Apathy

Apathy is the loss of motivation. It can manifest as someone no longer going out or engaging in activities they used to enjoy. Apathy is often one of the earliest symptoms of dementia. It can be hard to tell the difference between this and depression.

Emotional lability

Emotional lability can lead to rapid changes in mood. People with dementia can show changes in how they express and experience emotions. Sometimes they can have a facile response to things that should be upsetting, such as laughing when they are unable to perform tasks on a cognitive assessment. Some people will go between laughing and crying for no discernible reason.

Language problems

The specific area of the brain that generates language is Broca's area, which is in the frontal lobe of the dominant hemisphere. When people have a type of dementia that impacts this part of the brain, they have significant trouble finding words, even familiar ones. (The fancy name for this inability is "logopaenic aphasia.") People with damage to this part of the brain might also experience more subtle changes, including a reduction in vocabulary or less ability to generate fluid speech. Some will rely on automatic phrases. When people have relatively preserved speech—in other words, they sound okay—it can actually mask the severity of other cognitive deficits.

Getting lost

We all carry a mental map within us of the places we know. People with dementia can lose this sense and get lost going to familiar places, even driving to the local shops. Many people with advanced dementia in residential care can struggle to remember which room is theirs. They can also lose their ability to understand the spatial relationships of objects, including themselves, which can contribute to an increased risk of falls.

Sleep disturbance

People with dementia often have difficulty sleeping. They can experience disturbance of the sleep–wake cycle and so wake up numerous times during the night. People with more advanced dementia can become disoriented at night and think it is morning, then go about their morning routine, waking anyone nearby. Sleep disturbance can also be an early symptom of dementia, and even precede other symptoms. Some people with dementia will have extremely vivid dreams that can be distressing to them and the person they share a bed with.

Difficulty with complex tasks

One of the key things I ask when I am assessing someone for dementia is whether they are having difficulty doing things they used to be able to do. This will differ for each person depending on their social role and preferred hobbies. For an artist, losing the ability to make art is relevant; for a cook—like Rose—it might be a decline in the ability to prepare a meal.

Psychiatric symptoms

Some people will develop delusions, paranoia, and hallucinations. These can be extremely distressing to the person with dementia and cause great difficulty for the caregiver. A person with dementia may believe their spouse is being unfaithful or they may refuse to let caregivers in the house because they believe the caregiver will hurt them or steal from them. It is relatively common for people with dementia to believe that others are stealing from them when they lose things. Some people with dementia can also have visual hallucinations. These don't always cause significant distress—some people see family members or little children, and they like their hallucinations.

Giuseppe

The first time Maria saw Giuseppe she was fourteen and wearing her school uniform, but when he smiled at her there was something in his eye that made her feel like a grown-up woman.

After that, to her the boys her age seemed just that: boys. He was ten years older, a real man, but he said she was too young. Still, every Friday, they would meet after school and he would buy her a gelato and they would walk and talk.

When Giuseppe decided to leave Italy and go to Australia, he asked her to wait for him. He said he would send for her when he was settled. He got a job at the Ford factory. It was good pay, but he told her he wouldn't send for her until he had bought her a house. He told her to train as a seamstress, as there would be work for her too. She started taking evening classes in English.

Finally, when she was nineteen, the letter came to say he had bought a house. Her father said an unmarried woman could not travel alone so, as she stood in the church, repeating her vows, she tried to imagine it was Giuseppe standing beside her, not her brother acting as his proxy.

When she got off the boat in Australia, the sun had the familiar heat and crisp light of home, but everything else was different. Giuseppe was proud of his car and the orange brick house he had bought for them. They drove through endless suburbs, house after house on isolated blocks. In the evening, when they went for a walk, there was no one around to talk to. At night, after Giuseppe was asleep, Maria wept for her family, for the way everyone in the village would come out at night. She wept for the place that she knew would never be home again.

The first day Giuseppe took her to the shop where she would sew, she found a new sense of belonging. The other women were Italian like her, and they embraced her in the Italian way that Maria had missed from home. Maria was pleased when the boss said that she could be the one to work with customers because she could speak some English. Over time, Maria found that her English improved.

When the babies came, she took the sewing home. Maria did what her mother had taught her and looked after Giuseppe, always putting him first, making his favorite foods and looking after the children. He was the head of the house, he loved her, and she loved that she made him happy.

When Giuseppe turned sixty-five and stopped working, so did Maria. In the first year they took a trip back to Italy, but when Maria suggested it again Giuseppe said it was too much. They joined the Italian club and saw friends, and Maria's life felt full, especially with her grandbabies. Then Giuseppe started to lose interest in going out. He wanted to stay home, and he wanted Maria to stay home and look after him. She would go to visit her friends, but Giuseppe would call wanting a coffee, a snack, or to change the TV channel. She had always obeyed him; she could not change now. He did nothing but sit and wait for her to serve him.

Maria knew that something was not right. She took him to doctor after doctor, trying to find out what was wrong. She needed to know why he wouldn't go out and why he would do nothing but sit in his chair.

When the doctor asked if she'd thought that maybe he had dementia, Maria was furious. She called her daughter as soon as she could, expecting the same response, but her daughter was silent. In that moment, Maria knew the doctor was right. Maria had spent her life serving Giuseppe and making him happy while he led the family. What was she supposed to do now?

Do men have different symptoms of dementia?

One of the challenges of diagnosing dementia in men is that for many older men (and some younger ones), part of their social role is to be served by their wife. This means that there might be very little in the way of practical tasks for them after retirement. It can also mean that when the main symptom is apathy, a dementia diagnosis can come quite late, because a wife will have compensated for her husband.

Most people think of dementia as forgetting, but the earliest symptom for many men (and women) is often apathy, which people don't recognize so easily. In a study of 2,809 people who were referred to a specialized memory clinic because of cognitive concerns, men were more likely to present with apathy than women. When women have heart attacks, they often present with symptoms different to the central crushing chest pain we associate with heart attacks. Women's symptoms are described as "atypical" and easily missed. Similarly, if apathy is considered atypical, and not as well recognized as a symptom of dementia as forgetting, dementia diagnoses in men can be missed, making the condition appear to be more common in women.

In the study mentioned above, men were also alive for less time than women after diagnosis, which relates to the earlier point about women being more likely to reach very old age, when dementia risk rises, and surviving longer after a diagnosis. If women are just more likely to be diagnosed, it would go a long way toward explaining why there are more women alive with dementia than men.

"I'm losing my mind"

When someone comes to see a doctor because they are experiencing memory loss, it does not mean they have dementia. Many people worry when they notice that their memory is not working as well as it used to. We call this "subjective memory loss." Subjective memory loss is a distressing experience, and it is worth considering whether there are contributing factors such as lack of sleep, medications someone is taking, or anxiety, which can be fixed. It is definitely worth seeing your doctor if you are worried about memory loss.

In a summary analysis of various longitudinal studies of people with ages around seventy, those with self-reported memory loss did show a slightly higher risk of developing dementia, but the risk was still very small at around 2 percent a year. This means that the vast majority of people worried about their declining memory don't develop dementia.

Menopause, brain fog, and dementia

Women spend around four decades having periods. I think most of us remember the momentous time of puberty, with all the outward and inward changes from the hormones rushing around us. This is also a time of great change for the brain. We need to acknowledge that the hormone changes of menopause, when the ovaries stop producing estrogen and progesterone, are just as significant.

Estrogen is thought to have an important impact on memory and learning. When a woman is pregnant, some hormonal brain remodeling seems to prepare her for the rapid period of new learning that comes in early motherhood.

Menopause is defined as the permanent cessation of ovarian function. Clinically, this is defined as going twelve months without a period.

Perimenopause starts about four years before menopause, and with the fluctuations in hormone levels, many women experience symptoms that include hot flashes and insomnia. Around two-thirds of women describe experiencing cognitive difficulties—or brain fog—around the time of the menopause transition. This can involve trouble remembering words or names or walking into a room and forgetting why they are there.

A subjective change in function is distressing, but looking at the research, it is very difficult to know how much of this translates to an actual decline in cognitive function. Many studies are cross-sectional (one-off surveys that capture only a moment in time), so they can't prove causation. In one cross-sectional study of 130 women, no difference in cognitive testing between women who were pre-, peri-, or post-menopausal was seen, but perimenopausal women did report higher dissatisfaction with their memory. Interestingly, women with more symptoms, like hot flashes, as well as a more negative attitude to menopause, reported more dissatisfaction with their memory.

Some people have suggested a causal association between brain fog around the time of menopause and women's higher incidence of dementia than men but, overall, there just isn't enough evidence to show that women have a significant drop in cognition, and there are also a lot of confounding factors.

Brain functions such as short-term memory and attention are very sensitive: As I have been at pains to point out, one night of very bad sleep will impair your short-term memory. Women around the age of fifty also usually have an awful lot going on in their lives. Anyone juggling a job, financial stress as retirement approaches, teenage children, and aging parents might feel their brain is overloaded and experience insomnia.

Brain fog around menopause is real and distressing, but it's also important not to give people the message that this is the beginning of dementia. It in no way means you are facing an irreversible decline. To definitively answer the question of whether brain fog in menopause is a risk for dementia, we really need studies with enough people—men and women—that run for long enough and that also measure other confounders, such as insomnia or depression, or even smoking. In the meantime, if you have brain fog, it is definitely worth seeing your GP to look for underlying conditions, and to discuss hormone replacement therapy and aspects of your lifestyle that could make a difference.

Orla

Orla's back was so painful. Every time she went for a walk with her husband, Frank, she had to stop and have a rest. She was leaning more and more on her frame, which was making it hard to spend time in her beautiful garden. Orla was also living with mild dementia, but she could still reheat meals, do some housework, and shower and dress. Orla and Frank went to see a surgeon about her back pain, who told them he could do an operation.

When Frank went to see Orla after the operation, she was asleep. She woke up, but she had no memory of why she was in the hospital. When the physiotherapist came to take her for a walk, she was again too sleepy. Later that day, Orla tried to get out of bed by herself and fell. After this, she was put in a bed near the nurses' station so they could watch her more closely, but this meant that there was noise at night.

Over the next few days, Orla continued to refuse to get out of bed in the day but was awake at night. Because she spent so much time in bed she also developed pneumonia, which was treated with antibiotics.

Eventually, Orla made it to rehabilitation and started walking again, but she never made a complete cognitive recovery. Orla's pain was a little better for a while, but the cost was a permanent worsening of her dementia.

Orla's experience demonstrates some of the risks and rewards we need to consider when treating older patients. When someone with dementia develops delirium, it can mean that they never return to the same level of cognitive function. The lesson is that it is really important to avoid delirium. In addition, people with dementia are at risk of poorer outcomes with surgery. Sometimes operations are unavoidable, but if the surgery is nonessential it is worth talking this through with a geriatrician to consider risks to cognition and other nonoperative management options.

Is it delirium or dementia?

As noted already, dementia usually progresses slowly. When someone suddenly becomes more confused, this can be a sign they have delirium.

I can only imagine delirium is like that moment between sleeping and waking when you wonder, "Where am I?" "What day is it?" but rather than quickly realizing you are safe in your own bed, next to your partner, you find you are in a strange and terrible place with pain, bright lights, and a stream of unrecognizable people asking questions like "Which day of the week is it?" Imagine a rising sense of panic when you realize you have no idea.

Delirium can be incredibly distressing. People can think that someone is trying to kill them or there is a conspiracy to keep them in prison.

Delirium is a sudden change in cognitive function where people have decreased attention and concentration. It can be precipitated by infection, medications, surgery, dehydration, sleep deprivation, pain, or even just a change in environment. There are two important considerations in delirium: the insult to the brain and how vulnerable that brain is. If the insult is bad enough, as with a head injury, anyone can get delirium. For people with a more fragile brain due to preexisting dementia, a small insult, like a new environment, can be enough of a stress to cause delirium.

In the hospital, we are unfortunately excellent at giving people delirium. We take people who are already sick, put them in a place with minimal natural light, give them medications that affect the brain, and wake them up multiple times a night. I certainly wouldn't be thinking straight the next day.

The most noticeable form of delirium is "hyperactive delirium," which is when people become agitated, confused, and hyperalert. There is often reversal of the sleep–wake cycle, with people drowsy during the day and awake at night. The less noticeable form, because people are not active, and which has a higher mortality, is "hypoactive delirium." This is when people become very sleepy. I can come to see a patient at ten in the morning, and they are difficult to rouse. They can then drift back to sleep while we are talking. In hospitals, when meals come at set times, this can lead to malnutrition because people can sleep through the mealtime. Many people will have a combination of hypoactive and hyperactive delirium.

When I see a patient with delirium, I try to look at easily reversible factors, like anything that could be causing pain or discomfort, or a new medication. My team and I try to reorient people and create an environment with natural light. Having a loved one there to help keep the patient calm and encourage food and fluid is also helpful.

Delirium is not a benign condition. People with delirium have a higher mortality rate in the hospital and over the next year. A substantial number have ongoing symptoms even twelve months later. Some people never recover to their previous level of cognitive function.

One important study highlighted this by recruiting 1,510 people, with a median age of seventy-seven, who were well. The study performed a baseline cognitive assessment of the participants and then followed up with them over the next two years. If they were admitted to the hospital during this time, they were assessed for delirium. People without dementia at the beginning of the study were protected against delirium, and if they did develop a delirium, it was usually less severe. People with normal cognition who did develop a severe delirium also had the biggest decline in cognition at follow-up. They also had a higher risk of death over the two years of the study.

We don't know what exactly is going on in the brains of people with delirium, but it does seem like it can leave a person with permanent damage.

The biggest risk factor for delirium is having preexisting dementia. For some people, an episode of delirium will be the first time it becomes apparent to the people who love them that there is something very wrong.

When does cognitive decline become dementia?

I do a lot of work with hospital inpatients—people who have unexpectedly found themselves sick in the hospital with an infection, or because of a fall, or because their care needs have suddenly increased beyond what their family can provide, which we call functional decline. Many people I meet have cognitive impairment, and my team and I need to find out if this is new or preexisting. When I speak to the people who know the patient well, I often find out that the person has had memory problems, or trouble with complex tasks and organization, over the course of years. The family have been able to help them, so it wasn't an issue.

In the next chapter, you'll learn about all the different tests that are part of the diagnostic workup for dementia, but what I want you to keep in mind is that symptoms always need to be considered in the context of the person. For some families, a woman's short-term memory loss will be a major problem; another family will consider it part of aging. Maybe they are both right. If you consider a man with significant apathy, who no longer initiates cooking or cleaning, whether he lives alone or with extended family will have a big impact on how much of a problem this symptom is.

To complicate this further, there are many different symptoms that can present in many orders. Some symptoms, such as severe paranoia, are more obvious, but others are subtle. If the cognitive changes are impacting someone's ability to get through day-to-day life, this is the time to consider that they might have dementia and need to see a doctor.

QUESTION 3:

How does a doctor diagnose dementia?

When someone is told they have a progressive terminal neurological disease it should seem life-changing. The thing is, getting the label isn't necessarily the life-changing part. A label is often just that: a label. By the time most people are diagnosed with dementia, the symptoms would have started long ago.

Most, but not all, people I see for cognitive assessment are there because someone who knows them well has concerns. These concerns usually relate to a very noticeable change, something that has made them worry. Some caregivers want help and to access services; many want to know if there is a treatment. Some people will seek the diagnosis of a loved one early; others put it off for as long as possible because they don't want to believe that it is really happening.

It is very important that the person with symptoms of dementia has someone who knows them well accompany them through the diagnostic process. This person can often help to describe the symptoms, and their trajectory, and provide practical and emotional support, especially if the patient has memory problems.

The first step

For someone with memory concerns, the best person to see first is the usual family doctor. They will be able to do blood tests to rule out conditions that mimic dementia, for example, low thyroid function, as well as some initial cognitive assessment with some cognitive screening questions, like the previously mentioned MMSE.

The family doctor will usually have known a patient over a long period of time, and therefore have some knowledge of the person's past medical history and their social supports. Often it will fall to the family of the person to bring up any problems with the doctor, as the person with symptoms may not do so. Some people with dementia will be very capable at masking memory deficits, and it may not be apparent in a routine medical appointment.

The type of workup needed will differ according to the age of the patient, their comorbidities, and other conditions, as well as the rapidity of cognitive change. Someone who has a very sudden change in cognition needs more urgent attention, particularly if they are relatively young, to ensure there is nothing reversible happening. For someone who is older, with a very slow symptom onset over years, there is often no harm waiting a few months to see the specialist.

There are many different specialists who may be involved in diagnosing someone with dementia. Some people will go to see a neurologist, others to a geriatrician, and some to a specialized memory clinic. Again, your family doctor will be best suited to recommend the right specialist in your area.

The doctors you might meet on your dementia journey

Family Medicine Doctor—since there are so many things that can cause cognitive decline, a family medicine specialist who knows the patient well is the best person to see first.

Neurologist—a neurologist is a specialist in diseases of the brain and nervous system.

Geriatrician (my job)—a specialist in older adults and conditions that are commonly associated with aging, which naturally include dementia.

Neuropsychiatrist—a psychiatrist that treats psychiatric problems as they relate to neurological conditions.

Psychiatrist of old age—a psychiatrist who specializes in older adults.

Visiting the specialist

One of the most important skills for any doctor is taking a clinical history. This means asking the right open questions, developing a rapport with the patient and their family member (or carer), then asking further focused questions and testing a hypothesis. The way I approach this is to get to know my patient. How do they define themselves? What do they do all day? I ask about education, work, retirement, hobbies, and friends. When I feel I have a good sense of my patient, I move into what has changed. This history needs to be specific to the person's life, to their own social role. For a woman who runs a household, it may be that she can no longer cook a lasagna from scratch. For a man who has never cooked lasagna in his life, being unable to do this is irrelevant. Since dementia is defined by an inability to perform a social role, everyone will be different.

I also listen carefully to the details someone gives me, what they leave out, and the type of language they use. Do they answer my questions in superficial ways? Do they give only vague, nondescriptive pictures of their lives—for example, answering "this and that" when I ask what their job was?

Even when I first meet a person who clearly has cognitive impairment, and I might suspect that they have dementia, I still need to find out whether this is a new state or not. If someone was perfectly well yesterday and today is terribly confused, this needs urgent investigation. If someone is confused and their family says that this is their normal state and they have had memory problems for years, I can take more time to make the diagnosis.

Cognitive tests

These are tests of memory and thinking that will look at different brain processes and how well they are working. They can include such things as remembering three words, making a subtraction, or drawing a clock. Two commonly used tests are known as the Mini-Mental State Exam (MMSE) and the Montreal Cognitive Assessment Score. For some people, this will be enough to definitively identify cognitive deficits; others will need further assessment.

Neuropsychology Assessment

If a specialist or geriatrician suspects someone has dementia, yet they still perform well on simple screening tests, the next step is neuropsychological testing. This is performed by a psychologist who has done additional training in cognitive assessment. It is a highly specialized role. Neuropsychologists diagnose many conditions in younger and older people, including autism, ADHD, and intellectual disabilities, and can take conditions such as these, as well as education levels, into account in their testing and diagnoses of dementia. For people with suspected dementia, a neuropsychologist will start asking about the cognitive symptoms, daily activities, and background of the person, such as education and work. They follow this with tests of various cognitive functions, including memory, attention, speed of thinking, and reasoning. Sometimes, especially if the diagnosis is uncertain, the testing will need to be repeated, perhaps a year later, to see if the person's cognitive skills have stayed the same or declined. A neuropsychological assessment can be extremely helpful to determine a pattern of cognitive deficits and so help greatly with the diagnostic process.

Neuropsychological testing can also identify strengths that might help a person compensate for areas of cognitive decline. It is just as important to identify these as any weaknesses.

A neuropsychological assessment can take around three to four hours, and the neuropsychologist can spend hours more writing their report. The neuropsychologist may also discuss the results with the person and their family and provide a written summary. They can also work with the person and their family to come up with strategies to support the person's cognitive skills.

Biomarkers and brain scans

There are two types of brain scans that we use to look for structural changes to the brain. A CT (computed tomography) scan is like a really strong X-ray. It can identify big changes, such as those caused by a stroke some time in the past or brain shrinkage, but it can also miss a lot of things. Magnetic resonance imaging, or MRI, gives us much more detail. MRI looks at structures in the brain, such as the size of the hippocampus and blood-vessel health. It can also pick up other causes of cognitive decline, such as a brain tumor. While MRI can show if there are changes in brain structure, it doesn't tell us about brain function.

Another test that can look at brain activity is a PET (positron emission tomography) scan. This measures metabolic activity in the brain by looking at how much glucose different parts of the brain are taking up. Someone's brain can look structurally normal on MRI, but a PET scan can show reduced activity in certain areas. This can also help to differentiate different causes of dementia.

Sometimes the doctor will also recommend a lumbar puncture. This involves sticking a needle into someone's spinal canal to extract fluid, which sounds worse than it actually is. A lumbar puncture can rule out other conditions that might cause cognitive decline, such as infections. It is also possible to look for biomarkers to indicate a buildup of abnormal proteins in the brain.

Actually, it's not dementia

Some people will go through the entire assessment process and leave without a diagnosis of dementia. Over the years ahead, their cognition will remain stable, and it will become apparent they don't have dementia at all. This is particularly true for people who are alcohol dependent and who decide to become abstinent. Since the alcohol is doing the damage, many people become stable or even improve when they no longer drink.

There are other people who seek help for memory concerns who are actually undergoing an extremely stressful time in their life. They can become more forgetful under the strain because of reduced attention, and can be irritable and withdrawn. Some people will improve when a stressful life event is resolved or by finding strategies to manage anxiety.

As Brett's story below shows, coming away without a label of dementia can cause a wrench within a family as great as a diagnosis *of* dementia. People have excused behaviors and adjusted their expectations and social roles accordingly. Finding out that their loved one doesn't have a progressive terminal neurological disease should be a relief, but instead it throws an entire family dynamic into question.

Brett

For years, Brett's family had been tiptoeing around him. They knew they had to be extra careful not to do or say anything that might set him off. Brett had worked as a forklift driver, but he lost his job when he was forty-five after he nearly ran over another worker. After being reprimanded, he then called his boss a racial slur.

Brett didn't try to get another job. His days had a regular rhythm. He would get up and walk the dog, then he would go into the living room and start watching TV. His wife Cheryl took on extra hours as a clerk at the hospital, and his children learned to get themselves dinner. The house grew increasingly tense. Brett's children stopped asking their friends to come over, as they never knew when their father would explode. Cheryl would come home from work and bring Brett his dinner, always pausing at the door, a sick feeling of not knowing whether he would call her a "stupid bitch" or just grunt when she walked in the room.

Cheryl looked up his symptoms online and felt an intense sense of relief when it all started to fit with dementia. Cheryl found it easier to cope with Brett's moods because now she knew they weren't his fault. Brett felt relieved too. He finally had an explanation for how he felt, a reason for the way he behaved. Cheryl and the children did everything they could to support Brett, because Brett didn't want to see a doctor. However, Cheryl was still struggling financially and hoped that Brett would qualify for disability support, so she took Brett to a specialist in diagnosis of younger-onset dementia.

Brett saw a psychiatrist and neuropsychologist and had blood tests and an MRI. After multiple sessions, he got his formal diagnosis: he didn't have dementia.

Cheryl walked out of the appointment stunned. She had turned everything in her life around to support Brett, spending years compensating and hiding in her own home. Now she learned it wasn't his disease—it was him.

What are the stages of dementia?

One of the defining features of dementia is that it progresses over time. During the initial stages, a person with dementia might experience symptoms such as apathy and memory problems but will usually be able to participate in everyday activities and do household tasks, such as housework and light meal preparation. As the disease progresses to a moderate stage, cognitive symptoms are more obvious, and people living with dementia can experience distressing symptoms like paranoia and agitation. This can be in response to unmet needs or difficulty integrating and acting on physical and sensory information. In advanced dementia, the person with dementia will lose the ability to undertake many everyday tasks including feeding themselves, walking, or toileting. At this stage a person will require twenty-four-hour care.

It might seem simple and straightforward that people should seek help in an early stage, but for many, there isn't significant caregiver stress at this point and therefore no perceived problem. Many families will see memory changes as a normal part of aging, and if the person with dementia isn't distressed and the family isn't distressed, is there really a problem? For others, early symptoms can cause significant distress to both the person experiencing the symptom and the caregiver.

While advanced dementia, when much function has been lost, is more easily defined, the boundaries between mild and moderate are much more fluid and will depend on the individual's symptoms, their usual life role, and the practical and emotional capabilities of the people around them.

Timely, not early, diagnosis

Professor Shaun O'Keeffe, an Irish geriatrician, says we should be aiming for timely diagnosis rather than early diagnosis. Giving someone a label of dementia, with the prediction of deterioration and death, and the associated stigma, can be a heavy burden. Living with the self-surveillance of a diagnosis of dementia, or mild cognitive impairment, constantly worrying about the future and spiraling with every mental slip, is no way to live. This is particularly true for people who are older and frail and already have a limited life expectancy. For this group, there is nothing to be gained from hours of intensive cognitive testing and brain scans. For frail, older adults with symptoms, who are still functioning well, a label is likewise not especially useful.

For some people, getting a dementia diagnosis will mean being able to trial treatments that may help with symptoms. A diagnosis can also be a trigger to having important discussions about things like advanced care planning and creating an enduring power of attorney, although ideally these are things all adults should have in place regardless of their health.

One major benefit of getting a diagnosis is that it means being able to get support. Some clinics will have education sessions to help the person living with dementia and their caregiver understand the condition.

A blood test to rule it out

One of the challenges in dementia is that to do good quality research, especially in the search for treatments that protect the brain at the earliest stages of damage, we need to be able to have a more standard approach to diagnosis.

My colleague, associate professor Rosie Watson, leads a laboratory that is working on an early diagnosis for dementia with a simple blood test. Over coffee, in the University of Melbourne's neuroscience building, she told me that if we don't develop a better way to diagnose dementia, we won't be able to develop effective treatments. Her work focuses on neurofilament light chains, which are the skeletons of cells. These can be detected in the cerebrospinal fluid (CSF) when there is damage to brain cells. Their presence isn't specific to one type of dementia; they demonstrate any kind of neuron damage and will also be detected with other causes, like the autoimmune disease multiple sclerosis or with a brain injury.

Where they are showing promise is distinguishing mental illness from dementia. If someone has schizophrenia or depression, there won't be neurofilaments in their CSF. If they have dementia, there will be. This has huge implications for prognosis and treatment.

Right now, these neurofilaments are only being looked at in the CSF, and getting this requires a lumbar puncture, but Rosie thinks that in future it will be possible to get results from a blood test. If neurofilaments are not detected, they can be reassured they don't have dementia.

Biomarker tests, which will improve the sensitivity and specificity of diagnosis, are really critical to understanding all the types of dementia.

What are the types of dementia?

When someone receives a diagnosis of dementia, it is quite likely that they will be told which particular disease they have that is causing dementia. This is based on the symptoms and signs, which we know correlate with certain types of damage to the brain, from studies of people who have had assessments while alive and donated their brain for autopsy after death.

This list of diseases is far from complete—there are over one hundred different diseases that can cause dementia. The majority of older people with dementia will have Alzheimer's disease/vascular dementia. As you will read in later chapters, there is also still a lot to learn about exactly what is causing the damage to the brain in these diseases.

Alzheimer's disease

This is the most common type of dementia and is believed to be caused by a buildup of amyloid, or abnormal proteins, outside the cell and clumps of proteins inside the cell (although, as you will read in the next chapter, this is controversial). The symptoms most commonly associated with Alzheimer's are rapid forgetting, but many people will also have other symptoms, like getting lost, or having trouble finding words, or difficulty in problem-solving.

It's usually Alzheimer's even if it's not Alzheimer's

In Australia, to get medications at a subsidized rate someone has to have a diagnosis of Alzheimer's disease, not any other type of dementia. This is because back in the 1990s, when trials of drugs were being undertaken, the diagnostic criteria for Alzheimer's were based only on clinical history. This meant that many people in the trial would have actually had other forms of dementia. Later studies of people with Lewy body disease and vascular dementia have shown that when they were treated with anticholinesterase inhibitors (see Question 10), their symptoms improved, but so far, in Australia, these drugs have only been approved for Alzheimer's disease. This means that if a clinician suspects a patient has Lewy body, they will be labeled as mixed Lewy body/Alzheimer's or mixed vascular/Alzheimer's so the patient can get the medication at the subsidized rate. To be fair, this is actually reasonable because the different disease processes are hard to tell apart clinically, and the doctor can't be completely sure about what is causing the damage without a brain autopsy.

This also means that in Australia there would be no way to use routine data on drug prescriptions to accurately estimate the number of people with each subtype of dementia.

Vascular dementia

Vascular dementia is caused by a blockage or hemorrhage in the blood vessels in the brain—that is, by strokes that lead to the death of parts of the brain because of lost blood supply. Sometimes strokes are large and obvious, leading to significant obvious deficits like losing the ability to move half the body; sometimes they are small and go unnoticed. It is not uncommon that we do a CT of an older person's brain for an unrelated reason and find evidence of an old stroke that didn't cause any noticeable symptoms at the time. Vascular dementia can progress in a stepwise fashion, with a sudden change in physicality, but it can also have a slow and insidious progression like Alzheimer's. People with vascular dementia may have relatively preserved memory, although recall can be slower, and they might have worsened executive function and demonstrate apathy. Almost everyone with dementia aged eighty and over will have a combination of vascular disease and amyloid plaques.

Lewy body dementia/Parkinson's disease

Lewy body dementia has a lot of crossover with Parkinson's disease; indeed, the label of Lewy body or Parkinson's usually depends on whether a person develops cognitive or motor symptoms first. People with Lewy body disease will often have memory loss, trouble with complex thought processes, visual hallucinations, and motor-system impairments such as a shuffling gait, rigidity, and tremors. While many people with Parkinson's, in which the motor-system impairments usually manifest first, have normal cognitive function, they are nevertheless at very high risk of developing dementia if they have had the disease over a long period. Parkinson's disease and Lewy body dementia are both caused by "Lewy bodies," which are another form of tangled-up protein called "alpha-synuclein," although these proteins are also present in the brains of some cognitively normal older people. People who develop Lewy body dementia almost all suffer sleep disturbance, often with vivid dreams. Cognition can fluctuate throughout the day, and visual hallucinations are relatively common; for some reason these are often little insects or ants. Parkinson's disease most commonly occurs in men.

Frontotemporal dementia (Pick's disease)

As its name suggests, this is a dementia that predominately affects the frontal and temporal lobes of the brain. It is recognized as a "tauopathy," which means that the brains of people with frontotemporal dementia have accumulation of "neurofibrillary tangles" similar to the ones seen in Alzheimer's disease. People with this kind of dementia usually develop symptoms, such as apathy or an inability to organize or become disinhibited, which are associated with frontal lobe damage. Some people develop an overwhelming preference for sweet foods. Others develop language problems. Rarely do people develop motor symptoms, and very few will have motor neuron disease. The average age of diagnosis of frontotemporal disease is in the fifties. There is an inherited form of frontotemporal dementia, and so some people with FTD—and their families—may need genetic counseling.

Progressive supranuclear palsy (PSP)

This is a rare disorder that comes from damage to the cerebral cortex and an area called the "midbrain," which regulates movement and is located deep inside the brain. People develop a combination of rigid muscle tone and postural instability, with falls and cognitive dysfunction with particular frontal lobe involvement. The name comes from a loss of eye movement. People with PSP have trouble moving their eyes to look up and down or to smoothly track objects as they change position in front of them. Like FTD, it is a tauopathy, but the neurofibrillary tangles are structurally different, and of a different shape from those seen in Alzheimer's disease.

Corticobasal degeneration

This is a rare condition that leads to dementia as well as changes in movement. People can develop rigidity, increased muscle tone, and cognitive problems. They can also develop apraxia, or difficulty with a learned motor sequence, such as brushing their teeth, although this will often only affect one side of the body. Some people will develop alien limb syndrome, whereby their arm will seem to be acting of its own accord. Corticobasal degeneration is also a tauopathy.

Juliette

As a girl, Juliette loved nothing better than to draw and paint. At dinner time, her parents were always urging her to eat: Otherwise she was too busy creating art with her peas and mashed potato. By the time she was a teenager she had a job at the local art gallery, helping with stock and some light cleaning. Juliette learned she didn't just love art; she loved artists. She had an incredible eye for talent and what would sell. Many years later, when the gallery owner retired, Juliette took a deep breath, and a deep bank loan, and bought the gallery.

With her uncanny knack for spotting up-and-coming artists, and the fact that everyone knew she threw extremely good parties, the gallery thrived. Anyone who was anyone (at least with enough money) would come to her to get the best new piece to display their excellent taste.

Juliette promised that the day she turned sixty-five she would retire. She wanted to spend her days seeing all the art she had never yet seen.

It was when she was traveling in New York, walking through the Metropolitan Museum of Art, that her lifelong friend Javier noticed something was very wrong: Juliette couldn't recognize any of the pictures. Once Javier noticed this, he noticed other things, like Juliette's trouble with reading and that she was struggling to safely cross roads. Javier and his husband were worried enough that they flew back home with Juliette and took her straight to the doctor.

Juliette had a rare variant of Alzheimer's disease called "posterior cortical atrophy." In this case, the disease process was focused in the occipital lobes. While her eyes worked perfectly well as a sensory organ, she couldn't make sense of the information coming in. This also impacted her ability to read and safely navigate the world, but her memory was relatively preserved. The special ability that had defined her life, her ability to spot art, was the very one that was taken from her first.

Alcohol dementia

This is something I see far too commonly. Alcohol is a direct toxin to the brain. People with dementia from alcohol often have damage to the hippocampus and frontal lobes, which can lead to poor judgment, personality change, and trouble remembering. People often think of excess alcohol as a problem for the young, but I have seen many older adults who drink too much. Often, someone who has been drinking over a long period will develop memory problems. They can forget how many glasses of alcohol they have had, and so drinking escalates. Someone who was in the habit of drinking two large glasses of wine every night starts finishing a bottle, and over time the damage accumulates. This is why it is very important to not get into the habit of regular alcohol intake. It is just too easy for this to escalate. If this brings up concerns for you, I strongly suggest seeing your doctor.

Chronic traumatic encephalopathy

Chronic traumatic encephalopathy (CTE) is caused by repeated head trauma and has been recognized for a long time in the medical community. The other name for it is "dementia pugilistica," or more colloquially being "punch drunk." It's not completely clear what severity of head trauma is needed to cause CTE. Football including soccer, rugby and rugby league, American football, and Australian Rules have all had players affected by it. This has led to changes in the rules of some sporting codes, especially when it comes to concussion management, with some governing bodies introducing mandatory time off after a concussion.

Davey

The Glasgow Gorbals was where you lived when you had nowhere else to go, so after Davey's dad lost his job, this is where they went. Davey couldn't remember his dad before the war, but his mom said he was kind, patient, and gentle. Never touched the bottle. After the war it was different. When Davey's dad was good, he was the best dad in the world. He would help Davey with his reading and kick the soccer ball with him all day long. But then the dark would come to him. Davey would come home from school and smell the booze before he saw his dad. Sometimes his dad would have passed out, but sometimes he would be pacing with rage, and Davey knew then that he needed to protect himself and his brothers from a beating. Davey would grab his little brothers and take them to the soccer club, where at least they could get warm and sometimes get a meal.

The coach of the club took Davey under his wing. Twice a week, Davey would practice. He was fast, precise, and doggedly determined. His specialty was the header, and he would practice this over and over. When he was fourteen, Davey left school and went down the mines, but he kept playing soccer. He eventually became the coach and made it his mission to help other boys in similar circumstances to his own.

Davey did his best to stay out of trouble, but sometimes, after a few too many drinks he would get into fights outside the pub. He was known for his toughness and ability to keep standing, even after a few blows to the head. Fighting was also a good way to make an extra pound or two when he bet on himself.

One thing Davey was proud of was that he was not like his dad. His wife, Gwen, loved that he was such a kind and gentle man, so when Davey was in his fifties and started having outbursts of rage, his family was worried.

Davey would forget where he put things, then he would get angry with Gwen, accusing her of stealing. He started shuffling when he walked. Once he accused Gwen of having an affair and cornered her, so Gwen fled to her daughter's house, terrified.

After seeing a neurologist, Davey was diagnosed with dementia.

Davey's story is not unique among soccer players, who have a higher risk of dementia than the general population because of repeated, mild concussions from heading the ball. Along with the punches to the head, Davey suffered damage that sadly led to cognitive decline in a way that was devastating to him and his family.

QUESTION 5:

Do we actually know what causes Alzheimer's?

"Disease" is a confusing term. A disease is a label, a diagnosis given by a doctor, based on clinical assessment. Alzheimer's disease means that a doctor of some sort believes that the person has signs and symptoms that indicate there is a particular type of damage in the brain. Alzheimer's disease is only diagnosed when there is enough dysfunction or damage to cause signs or symptoms.

For the disease gout, when someone has a painful, red-hot swollen joint, we can stick a needle in, and a pathologist can look at the fluid under a microscope to see crystals with a particular shape. For dementia, we do not have such a simple way to link the molecule causing the mischief to what a person is experiencing. A disease label is an attempt to link physiology and cell function to symptoms and prognosis, and ideally to treatment.

For decades, the theory of Alzheimer's has been that a molecule called amyloid is the cause of the brain damage, but increasingly, doctors and researchers are not so sure. You might have seen the word "amyloid" come up a few times now. Amyloid refers to fragments of protein that form clumps outside cells in our body. These clumps are called "fibrils" because when scientists use a certain stain to look at them under the microscope, they appear a similar color to the fiber that forms the outer layer of plant cells. While proteins in our body can do all sorts of things, such as form structures or enzymes that catalyze chemical reactions, or act as the gates to entry into a cell, these clumps of amyloid do nothing useful (as far as we know right now). Primary amyloidosis, which can cause liver and kidney failure, has been known about since the mid-1800s.

In 1906, the psychiatrist and neuropathologist Alois Alzheimer peered through his microscope at slices of brain from a deceased patient, Auguste Deter, whom he had treated for what was then known as "presenile dementia." He identified the microscopic changes that have come to define the disease that bears his name. For the next few decades, people thought Alzheimer's disease was rare. It wasn't until the 1960s that pathologists started to notice that a buildup of plaque was common in older adults that had been diagnosed with dementia before they died.

While Alzheimer had identified the amyloid plaques in the brain, it was in the 1980s that further critical discoveries were made. In 1984, George Glenner and Caine Wong, working at the University of California at San Diego Medical School, published a paper describing the sequence of the protein that made up the amyloid plaques. They hypothesized that amyloid could be derived from a precursor that circulated in the blood. In 1985, Professor Colin Masters at the University of Melbourne and his collaborators published a paper describing the cerebral amyloid found in dementia patients. This work led to the amyloid hypothesis: the idea that the buildup of amyloid is the cause of Alzheimer's disease.

The amyloid precursor protein discovered by Glenner and Wong sits in the cell membrane and seems to have multiple important functions, although no one is entirely sure what they all are. Amyloid seems to have a role in the function of brain synapses and helping neurons communicate with one another. Certain enzymes cleave (or cut) the part of the protein that sticks out of a cell, and this releases amyloid-beta, which is a fragment of amyloid-precursor protein. Amyloid-beta (a-beta) can bind to other chaperone proteins (including APOEe4) and then be removed from the brain into the blood, where it travels to the liver or kidneys to be broken down.

Depending on where the protein is cleaved, these amyloid-beta protein fragments vary in length. All amyloid-beta will clump together, but longer fragments clump more readily and are insoluble. The accumulation of amyloid is caused by overproduction or a lack of removal.

The amyloid hypothesis for dementia is that it is these clumps that cause all the damage, including cell death and synapse dysfunction, that leads to what we see in an Alzheimer's death.

Alongside the amyloid plaque is another protein called "tau." Tau is normally a structural protein found inside neurons; it acts like scaffolding. In Alzheimer's disease, the tau proteins show chemical changes that make them tangle up. Studies in mice have shown that tau usually develops after amyloid, and so the theory is that the amyloid plaques drive the development of tau.

The arguments for amyloid

One of the earliest pieces of evidence that amyloid was the culprit in Alzheimer's disease came from genetic studies. Inherited forms of Alzheimer's disease make up less than 5 percent of all cases, and around 60 to 70 percent of all younger onset cases. Sixteen different gene mutations have been identified that cause inherited Alzheimer's disease. These gene mutations are fully penetrant, which means if you have them, you are guaranteed to get the disease. Many of these genes are involved in cleaving proteins, which can result in the amyloid precursor protein being cut in a spot that leads to formation of the "a-beta" form of amyloid.

Other people have mutations in the gene that codes for the amyloid precursor protein. This gene is located on chromosome 21. Another piece in the genetic puzzle is that people with Down syndrome, who have three copies of chromosome 21, so three normal copies of the gene for the amyloid precursor protein, have extremely high rates of Alzheimer's disease by the fifth decade of life, although it is worth noting that even with this high amyloid burden, dementia is not universal.

As mentioned previously, until relatively recently, the only way to know whether someone had amyloid in their brain was via an autopsy after death. Amyloid PET has changed that. An amyloid PET scan is a brain scan that involves injecting a special tracer into the patient's blood, which "sticks" to amyloid in the brain and shows up on the scan, enabling researchers to measure how much amyloid is present.

Currently, amyloid PETs are only used in the research setting. The Australian Imaging, Biomarker & Lifestyle Flagship Study of Ageing (AIBL) was started in 2006 to study biomarkers, brain imaging, lifestyle factors, and dementia. Researchers recruited 333 cognitively normal people ranging between 60 and 89 years of age and followed them for 54 months, tracking changes in cognition and how this correlated with their amyloid load. At the beginning of the study, 84 people (25%) had a high amyloid load. Over time, 218 (65.5%) showed stable memory, 103 (30.9%) showed subtle decline, and 12 (3.6%) showed a rapid decline. To put that in perspective, the group with rapid decline reached this state 1.5 years after the trial started. If the study had continued, the researchers predicted that the group with "subtle" decline would have reached memory impairment at around 14 years after the trial started, although of course we cannot know that for sure. People with a positive amyloid PET were significantly more likely to be in the group with a rapid decline in memory.

This study is consistent with other studies around the world showing a link between positive amyloid PET and cognitive decline, but the problem is that correlation doesn't always equal causation. This principle is beautifully illustrated by a study published in the prestigious *New England Journal of Medicine*, which showed that countries where people ate more chocolate won more Nobel prizes. While we would all love to think that eating a lot of chocolate will make you a brilliant thinker, this is correlation, not causation. To take this back to the amyloid hypothesis, it is entirely possible amyloid is a mere bystander, a marker that something else is damaging the brain.

The arguments against amyloid

One of the major ways the argument for amyloid as a unifying hypothesis falls down is that it is just so common in older brains, with around half of all cognitively normal people having amyloid and a whopping 98 percent having tau tangles. To complicate this further, in adults ages eighty and older almost none have pure Alzheimer's pathology. They almost all have damage to blood vessels as well, meaning less blood supply to all or parts of the brain.

By the time two people have reached very old age, generally there have been a lot of different things about their lives: work, food choices, living circumstances, social engagement, and community support. These are variables that researchers like to eliminate when they study the causes of disease.

One way to minimize this variation is to study a group that has lived very similar lives, which is why a study with nuns is so illuminating. Participants in the nun study were all Catholic sisters born before 1917 and recruited between 1991 and 1993. The 678 participants had cognitive assessments taken when they were alive, and 38 had brain autopsies after death. Within this group of 38, who mostly died in their mid to late eighties, some were cognitively normal, some had mild cognitive impairment, and some had dementia. There were women in each of these groups with a significant amyloid load. Two nuns with the same amyloid load could have had a very different clinical picture.

Many researchers believe amyloid is important but not the only factor in explaining these discrepancies: It may be that there are multiple steps involved in the damage, so amyloid alone is not enough. One possible explanation is that there are two forms of amyloid, one that is soluble and one that is not, and researchers have postulated that only the soluble form causes damage.

Another clue comes from a study where researchers measured iron in people's brains using a special MRI. The study found that people with a high amyloid burden and a low level of iron in the brain had preserved cognitive function. It's important to note that the level of iron in the brain has more to do with the brain's own metabolic functions than iron in the diet.

The other aspect of this is tau, the protein tangles inside the neurons. Cognitive function is more strongly linked to tau burden than to amyloid. Tau distribution also maps closely to cognitive dysfunction and to brain atrophy. People with frontotemporal dementia, for example, show significant levels of tau even without amyloid plaques.

Mouseheimer's* or Alzheimer's?

Before the first dose of a new drug can be given to a human subject, it is tried out on animals. In the 1990s, when the amyloid theory became widely accepted, researchers needed a way to study it in laboratory animals. Since dementia is an age-related disease, and rats and mice live for only two to three years, they offer a much more manageable time frame for a study. The only problem was that, while some animals do accumulate amyloid in the brain with aging, animals don't seem to develop dementia the way humans do. In 1995, researchers were able to create a transgenic mouse that

---

* I did not make up the term "mouseheimer's," and I don't know who did.

developed amyloid plaques in its brain, then caused cognitive deficits by inserting a gene from a familial form of Alzheimer's disease. With further work, they were able to create a mouse that started developing plaques in its brain at only two months old.

Researchers have made excellent progress creating drugs that can cure dementia in transgenic mice, but these have not translated to cures for humans. Part of the problem is that the mouse models of dementia create amyloid plaques in a different way from humans. The mice also develop damage at a relatively young age, unlike humans, who usually develop dementia at an older age.

This brings up a fundamental difficulty in devising an animal model to research an age-related disease; we don't know why different animals age at different rates. In general, we can't automatically apply any knowledge gained from animal studies of aging to humans (despite what many self-described antiaging experts will tell you when they try to sell you a supplement).

No other animal, including nonhuman primates, are known to develop spontaneous Alzheimer's disease. While the brains of animals do change with age, they don't develop typical Alzheimer's pathology. So the next time you read a headline about a cure for dementia, then see that it is in mice, by all means, enjoy the science, but understand that this is far from a cure in humans.

Beware the sunk cost

Karl Popper, a philosopher of science, wrote that "whenever a theory appears to you as the only possible one, take this as a sign that you have neither understood the theory nor the problem which it was intended to solve."

One of the very real risks of the decades spent holding up amyloid as the one theory to unite them all is that there has been relatively little research into other possible causes of dementia. It is an extreme extrapolation that the genetic disease that impacts people in their forties is the same as the disease of people in their eighties and nineties. Trying to wrap everything into a unifying theory of amyloid ignores the overwhelming evidence about the importance of lifestyle, including exercise, nutrition, and cognitive impairment.

Research funding is incredibly competitive. Scientists can spend up to 50 percent of their time just writing grant applications to try to get funding and many of these won't succeed. They are incentivized to overextend and to overpromise that they, and they alone, have the answer. I don't blame anyone for wanting to write the most compelling grant application: they are literally fighting for their job. And it isn't true just of the people researching amyloid. I have read articles by researchers exploring other potential causes of dementia that discuss only their topic of interest to the exclusion of other theories.

Research is funded based on past success, so those that have come up with a novel and exciting discovery early in their career, and have built on that, have no incentive to change paths. The amyloid hypothesis is a hypothesis: an idea that we must test. The complexity of a disease like Alzheimer's means that we need to keep questioning and testing all its facets.

To be a scientist is to be uncertain. A scientist can spend their entire career focusing on one small corner of the universe, only to have another team come along and run an experiment that makes their theory redundant. The ideal scientist remains skeptical and holds tight to scientific integrity, ready to unemotionally give up a life's work to the higher cause of truth. Of course, scientists are human. Scientists are fallible and open to confirmation bias. Scientists have egos and want to leave a legacy. Scientists don't want to see a lifetime of work diminished. Yet, we can never know it all. We can never be completely confident we are right, but we can build on the knowledge that has come before.

There are other theories on what starts the damage in many types of dementia. As they are all caused by neurodegenerative processes, there may be some commonality in their beginning. In the next chapters, I will talk about what can go wrong in the ways our bodies operate and repair damage, starting with aging, the most common risk factor for dementia of all.

What is the role of aging in dementia?

When I occasionally look at a CT scan of the brain of someone in their twenties or thirties, I am struck by just how different it looks from the brain of someone in their eighties or nineties, like most of my patients. We can roughly tell someone's age by looking at them on the outside, and their brains look different too.

Aging is a complex biological phenomenon that results from many of the cellular processes that are essential to life. We will later examine social factors, which are hugely important, but right now it's time to look more deeply at cells and their role in our bodies. This means there will be more scientific terms ahead.

At the cellular level, there are four main contributors to aging: DNA damage, telomere shortening, epigenetic change, and mitochondrial damage.

All our cells, other than ova and sperm, contain twenty-three pairs of chromosomes, which are essentially bundles of deoxyribonucleic acid (DNA). DNA contains the instructions for our cells to make more copies of one another and to undertake all the complex chemical reactions that make life possible. When you get a Lego set, there are written instructions that tell you which pieces to put in which order, turning a random collection of blocks into an orderly creation. Similarly, the instructions in DNA tell the cellular building machinery which amino acids to put in which order to form proteins. The correct order of amino acids is very important for the protein to then fold into the right shape for its function, so if the DNA sequence isn't right, the protein won't be right. Proteins have many functions, including as the building blocks of cells, chemical messengers, and enzymes for chemical reactions.

Every time our cells divide, they make another copy of DNA, but this process is not perfect, and there will always be errors. While there are repair mechanisms within our cells, these won't catch every error, and so, the older we get, the more errors that accumulate. Some DNA errors won't impact cell function, but if an error occurs in a critical spot, it can have a huge impact. If an error impacts the production of an essential protein, the cell might not work. If an error occurs in a gene that impacts the regulation of cell division, it can start a cascade of errors that lead to cancer.

Another change that happens to our DNA with age is that telomeres, which are extra caps of DNA on the end of our chromosomes, get shorter. While we have enzymes to repair these, over time our telomeres inevitably shorten. When they become critically short, the DNA becomes so unstable that the cell will no longer divide.

Even in cells that don't make more copies of themselves, like neurons, DNA can still be damaged by other processes going on within the cell. As we get older, the repair mechanisms for this damage don't work as well as they once did, so cells accumulate increasing amounts of damage.

If you were to unwind DNA it would be around 2 meters in length, so most DNA is tightly wound up around proteins in what we call "DNA methylation." This also regulates which genes are switched on and which are not. With age, the patterns change in a predictable way, partly as a response to DNA damage. These are the epigenetic changes of aging.

Once a protein has been produced, it can also get damaged and need repair. When a protein is damaged so that it has lost its shape, it can also damage others around it, leading to a cascade of misshapen proteins. (This is part of the amyloid hypothesis: that amyloid itself creates more amyloid.)

Being alive, and all the essential chemical reactions that entails, uses an awful lot of energy, which we need to unlock from the food we eat, after it is broken down into molecules that can get into our cells. Inside our cells, small structures called mitochondria facilitate a controlled explosion between glucose and oxygen to unlock this energy, which is then used by the cell to power other chemical reactions to make things such as proteins. The energy released does not always go where it is supposed to and this is another way that cellular damage can occur, including to the DNA and the mitochondria themselves. Since the brain is so metabolically active, the mitochondria are at a high risk of damage. If there is enough damage, the cell will die. If there is less damage, the cell might become senescent.

A senescent cell can no longer divide or perform its normal function, but it still sends out chemical signals that influence what is going on around it. Sometimes these cells are described as zombies, but I don't think this captures the many helpful roles they still perform. Senescent cells have a role in wound healing, suppressing cancerous cells, and even embryonic development. Cells that divide, such as stem cells, can become senescent, and so can cells that don't divide, such as neurons.

Senescent cells can be cleared out by the immune system, but over a long life they accumulate, thereby having an impact on how well our immune system functions, which is critical for our health.

What is immunosenescence?

There are two times in life when we are particularly at risk from infections. The first is at the start of life, especially the first months after birth, when our immune system is underdeveloped. The second is after many decades of life. In older age, the accumulation of damaged cells and senescent cells means that the innate immune system is more active, leading to higher levels of nonspecific inflammation. We also have a decreased ability to produce antibodies, particularly to new disease-causing bacteria and viruses. This is why older adults need higher doses of many vaccines. At the same time, through the process of living and the accumulation of damaged cells, our immune system has more trouble turning off, leading to higher levels of inflammation, and this might actually be one of the key contributors to the damage to neurons that can cause dementia. This is discussed more in "Question 7: Does inflammation cause dementia?"

Frailty and dementia

Frailty is the loss of physiological reserve, which means someone is vulnerable to a significant decline from a seemingly minor insult. Frailty increases with age, but for people over sixty-five, frailty, rather than age alone, is actually a better predictor of mortality. By the time people are in their nineties, almost all have a degree of frailty. People with frailty are more likely to develop a disability.

Frailty is the result of age-related changes in our body. As the cellular damage accumulates over the course of living many years, our bodies become less efficient at utilizing energy and have to work harder to maintain "homeostasis," the state of being alive and in biological equilibrium. Since aging is associated with dementia, so is frailty. For the very elderly, it is false to try to separate the two, since they are part of the same process.

Why do women live longer than men?

A paradox of aging is that women are more likely to live longer than men, but with worse health and higher levels of frailty.

The reasons that younger men are more likely to die than younger women are heartbreaking: suicide and trauma. Men are more likely to do things that are risky; for example, drive while intoxicated. In younger old age, men are more likely to die from heart disease.

Women have some biological advantages. Women are less susceptible to infection than men, partly because the X chromosome has many genes to do with immune function. If you have only one X chromosome, you have fewer weapons in your immune armory. This is why women are more likely to survive infections than men.

The role of estrogen is also important. Prior to menopause, women have a much lower risk of heart disease than men, but after menopause they catch up. Further evidence for the cardioprotective effect of estrogen comes from women who have undergone early menopause, either due to premature ovarian failure or due to surgical removal of the ovaries. The earlier a woman goes through menopause, the more likely she is to have cardiovascular disease. Women who are prescribed estrogen after surgical removal of the ovaries prior to natural (later) menopause do not have an increased cardiovascular risk.

The association between cardiovascular health and menopause is exactly that: an association. It does not prove causation. It is entirely possible that the very same factors that lead to early menopause are part of the development of cardiovascular disease. As an example, cigarette smoking is a risk factor for early menopause and dementia, but not all studies take this into account.

The combination of protection against infection and decreased cardiovascular disease goes a long way to explaining why women have a longer life expectancy than men, but another important explanation comes from the countries where this gender life expectancy gap is narrowed: countries with high levels of equality between the sexes. This indicates that there is something about gendered social roles that can perhaps decrease the risk of early death for men.

As noted elsewhere, increased life expectancy also means women are more likely to live into very old age when dementia risk is highest.

How is the brain affected by aging?

Unlike most parts of the body, once we are adults we are not able to make any more brain cells (there is some debate about whether this is possible in the hippocampus, where some animal studies show that it is possible for neurons to keep dividing). This means that compared to other parts of the body, the brain is particularly vulnerable to a buildup of age-related change. These changes themselves can start to impact other critical brain functions, for example, the production of myelin, which means that neurons are much less efficient at transmitting signals to one another. All this damage, along with increased but less regulated immune signaling, can mean that the microglia become overwhelmed and struggle to repair the damage.

One real positive is that, while there are more people around with dementia because the population is getting older, the actual risk of dementia is declining, which is likely due to better control of cardiovascular risk factors and education. Just as there is a lot to be learned from studying disease, it is also worth studying those who remain well, to understand the protective factors, including psychosocial factors.

Aging is an inevitable part of living if you are lucky enough to live a long life. While dementia rates rise with age, dementia is not a normal part of aging. In fact, most people in their eighties and even nineties don't and won't have dementia.

QUESTION 7:

Does inflammation cause dementia?

I'm sure you can all relate to the experience of having the flu. You feel exhausted, your appetite is poor, you have trouble concentrating, your muscles ache, and you generally feel awful. These feelings aren't the virus: they are actually the by-products of the immune system springing into action. If you did a blood test, it would likely show high levels of inflammatory markers—the chemical signals our cells produce to put the whole body into action to fight the infection.

"Inflammation" has become something of a health buzzword because it is linked to so many chronic diseases, including diabetes, heart disease, and, now, dementia. One of the key findings in dementia research to date is that there seems to be evidence of overactivity of the brain's immune cells (the microglia mentioned a few times now) in dementia patients.

In the simplest terms, inflammation is activation of the immune system. The immune system is activated in response to bacterial or viral invaders, and it regulates the process of repairing damaged tissue and/or killing mutated cells that have become cancers. We can't survive without an immune system.

Inflammation is not binary—either on or off. Rather, the activity of the immune system exists along a spectrum, striving for a careful balance between fighting off continual threats but not so active that these same processes start to damage the very cells the system is supposed to protect. This is achieved by a constant interplay of chemical signals from immune cells in the body, meaning that inflammation is never truly confined to one part of the body.

How does the immune system fight off infection?

The immune system has two separate but very interconnected systems. The first is the innate immune system. When there is some kind of threat of infection, it is very important that the immune system is able to act quickly, and this is just what the innate immune system does. Our defenses against infection include barriers to bacteria and viruses getting in; these defenses include skin, tears, and snot. They also include first responder cells and chemical messengers called "cytokines." Let's pretend you were gardening and got a nail stuck in your foot. You would notice the pain and pull it out, but some dirt and bacteria would already have breached the skin. Sensing the tissue damage and bacteria, frontline immune cells called "neutrophils" and "macrophages" activate and start engulfing the debris. They send out chemical signals to draw more immune cells to the area and make the surrounding blood vessels leaky. This lets other immune cells into the damaged area, which then becomes warm, red, and swollen.

Innate immunity is quick and general. Humans are long-lived animals, and our immune systems have ways of learning from past experiences, through a process called "specific" or "humeral" immunity. These two components—the innate immune system and the specific system—intersect. Within the innate system, we have cells called "dendritic cells" and "macrophages." When they encounter a bacterial cell, they change shape to surround and engulf it. Enzymes are then produced that chop the bacteria into tiny pieces, which are then displayed on the surface of the macrophage. Bearing these offending particles, the macrophages travel through lymph vessels to the lymph nodes located in various places around your body—in your groin and armpits and in a chain along the inside of your abdomen. When the macrophages arrive, they look for a special antibody-producing cell that matches the bit of bacteria, virus, or other enemy they have on display. When they come across the perfect match, they link together like a lock and key, and turn on antibody production, making antibodies specific to that particular microscopic enemy. These antibodies then go out and attach to the foreign invader, making the invader cells an easy target for other immune cells to destroy.

If the invader cells are ones that the body has not encountered before, this process takes a few days to activate. If they are ones the body has seen before, antibodies are produced quickly and the infection is rapidly controlled. For instance, if it is the bacteria that cause tetanus that entered the body and you've had your tetanus vaccination within the last ten years, your body should be able to make a quick antibody response to the toxins produced by the tetanus bacteria and prevent you from becoming extremely sick.

Specific immunity is slower than innate immunity, but very effective. It means that if we have survived an infection or had a vaccine for it, our bodies will have memory of the enemy and can quickly act to fight it off again (although immunity can wear off over time).

What is the immune system of the brain?

Although it is protected, our brain is very much impacted by systemic inflammation and at risk of infection. As the command center, where all sensory information is received and interpreted to be appropriately responded to, it is important that our brains get a signal that there is a threat to survival. These signals are delivered by chemical messengers called "cytokines" and can lead to a spiking fever or that general achy, tired feeling you get when you have an infection. At the same time, to state the obvious, infection in the brain is very bad. Our bodies have many systems in place to try to protect the brain from invading bacteria, viruses, and other microbes, and there is also an extra layer of protection called "immune privilege." Due to a combination of physical barriers and immune system factors, the brain is somewhat sheltered from systemic inflammation and infection.

Since neurons are very busy cells and have high demands for nutrients and oxygen, they need an excellent blood supply. The cells that constitute the walls of blood vessels in the brain are bound together extra tightly, forming what is called the "blood–brain barrier." This limits the movement of cells in and out of the brain and provides a protective barrier. While peripheral immune cells can't move into the brain under normal conditions, the brain does have its own immune cells—the microglia we met in Question 2.

Microglia make up a surprisingly large proportion of brain cells, somewhere around 10 percent, and they are very busy cells. As well as fighting off pathogens, they help to keep the brain neat and tidy by repairing any damage, and even supporting neuronal function. Microglia can take different shapes and play different roles in various parts of the brain. In the hippocampus, they are more immune ready, which might be part of the reason the hippocampus is so vulnerable to damage from an overactive immune system.

Autopsy studies of people with Alzheimer's have shown microglia clustered around the amyloid plaques in the hippocampus. Many researchers believe that the accumulation of the abnormal plaques and tangles triggers activation of the immune system, which in turn causes damage.

One of the most important things to know about biology is that nothing is ever simple. It is gloriously complex—everything is interconnected. All physiological systems in our body impact one another, and this is particularly true of the immune system. Another thing to be aware of is that many scientists often disagree vehemently with one another. While some scientists believe that amyloid initiates the damage that leads to dementia, many others believe that increased inflammation is actually the initiating step.

During normal times, our microglia have a small central circle surrounded by tendrils that are looking out for any danger. Once they detect something abnormal, like damaged tissue or signs of infection, they change shape and become blob-like and mobile. The activated cells move to the danger site and can stay there for weeks. There they can either take on a defensive role, driving inflammation, called the "M1 phenotype," or take on a role in tissue healing, called the "M2 phenotype." The role they take on will depend on the cytokines—chemical messengers—around them, and they can change between the two roles. It is important that there is balance because too much inflammation can cause damage.

The chemical messengers that tell the cells to go into the M1 form are an important link with immune activity in the brain and inflammation in the rest of the body.

Inflammation should be a temporary phenomenon. If there is an imbalance between the on and off switches, in favor of on, especially over long periods of time, this can lead to damage and, eventually, disease.

Immune privilege also has its downsides. If a virus, bacteria, fungus, or even parasitic worm actually does get into the brain, it has a much better chance of evading the immune system and can stick around for a long time. If someone develops immune compromise, they can also develop a very severe brain infection. Some researchers believe that a common family of viruses, the herpes viruses, may even have a role in the development of dementia.

Herpes viruses

One of the pieces of evidence linking dementia and the immune system comes from intriguing links between herpes viruses and dementia.

The idea that herpes simplex virus 1 or 2 (HSV)—the virus that causes cold sores and genital herpes—could cause dementia has actually been around since the 1950s. Around 70 percent of people have been infected with HSV at some point in their lives, many without ever knowing they have had it. HSV sticks around forever in our bodies, hiding in nerve cells. This is why people can get regular recurrences of cold sores or genital lesions. Rarely, HSV can cause catastrophic infections in the brain with a high risk of death.

In a study done in Taiwan looking back at population health data, people over fifty with a new diagnosis of HSV were around 2.5 times more likely to then be diagnosed with dementia. While this study excluded people who had been diagnosed with HSV earlier in life, this doesn't mean that these were all new infections. I have made many "new" diagnoses of genital herpes in older adults who have not had a new sexual partner or even been sexually active for years. Theirs was not a recently acquired infection; it's just that the immune system becomes less good at controlling the infection with age, and people develop symptoms for the first time.

This study also pointed to a potential therapy: antiviral medication. Over ten years, in the group with HSV that didn't receive medication, 28.3 percent developed dementia. In the group that received medication, 5.8 percent developed dementia. This study was not a randomized controlled trial, so the results need to be interpreted with caution. It was also only looking at people with active HSV, not latent, so there may already be something different about this group that puts them at a higher risk of dementia.

Another study in Sweden has shown that people who have evidence of past HSV infection on a blood test have a higher risk of developing dementia.

Of course, this isn't an all-encompassing theory of dementia. This is an observational study, and it looks at correlation, not causation. Many people in the study who didn't have a new HSV diagnosis still developed dementia, and the people who had HSV also tended to have more medical problems, but it is certainly an area that merits further study.

How does inflammation impact the brain's function?

When you have the flu you don't feel like running a marathon. You have what is known as "sickness behavior," which means you want to crawl into bed and go back to sleep. For many people with autoimmune diseases, whereby the immune system becomes active against the body itself, fatigue can be one of the most disabling symptoms.

Anything that causes persistent systemic inflammation can increase brain immune-response activity and risk neurodegeneration. In a study of people with dementia, those who had episodes of high levels of inflammation, as measured on a blood test, had a more rapid cognitive decline. The study didn't talk about potential causes for the high inflammation; the blood test was simply a marker for high immune activity, which could be caused by many things (such as a viral or bacterial infection).

An intriguing hint about the role of systemic inflammation is that people with rheumatoid arthritis, an autoimmune inflammatory disease, have a degree of protection against dementia when placed on certain immune modifying drugs. There is also some evidence that giving people the kinds of anti-inflammatory medications called "nonsteroidal anti-inflammatory" drugs, such as ibuprofen, may decrease the risk of dementia, but we need more research to confirm this. For many older adults who have heart or kidney problems, these medications can also have significant side effects.

Does COVID-19 cause dementia?

One of the most alarming claims that has been repeated about COVID-19 infection has been that it causes dementia. In a study conducted in the UK, the authors made the claim that people who'd had COVID-19 were more likely to have cognitive decline than people of the same age who hadn't. There was a group in this study for which the evidence seems very strong: those who had been to intensive care. People who had been admitted to the hospital with COVID-19 also showed a higher incidence of dementia than those who had not had COVID-19, or who had experienced only a mild disease case.

There is nothing surprising in the fact that people who'd been very unwell had longer-term cognitive injury, because we've known for over a decade that people who spend a prolonged time in the ICU for respiratory failure often have persistent cognitive decline. We also know that people sick enough to get delirium won't make a full cognitive recovery. The risk factors for contracting a severe case of COVID-19, such as obesity, hypertension, and diabetes, are also the same risk factors for cognitive decline, and the study did not account for this.

Another widely shared study was a retrospective into a cohort, which recorded a higher incidence of many neurological illnesses, including epilepsy, psychosis, and dementia. This study relied on data that was collected as part of routine healthcare. It found that following a COVID-19 infection there was a higher incidence of a new diagnosis of dementia compared to other respiratory illnesses.

There are two problems with claiming causation in this study. The first is that a severe illness of any kind can lead to delirium and permanent cognitive decline, and this study did not account for disease severity; we know that COVID-19 is more serious than other respiratory illnesses. (Also, less than 5 percent of people in the study had been vaccinated against COVID-19, a statistic that was only visible in supplementary text, not the main body of the report. As a general rule, studies of disease severity in the pre-vaccine era can't be automatically applied to the post-vaccine era.)

The second is that when people come into contact with healthcare practitioners, they are then more likely to get unrecognized health problems diagnosed, such as dementia that had been manageable in the community before they got sick.

At the time of writing, the evidence is not strong enough to say that COVID-19 causes dementia. As someone with a science education, I can't say that we can rule it out either.

I don't want this to come across as dismissive. A new onset of cognitive decline is incredibly distressing, but it is absolutely not new knowledge that severe illness, with metabolic dysfunction, multiple organ failure, and an inflammatory storm, can have long-term consequences. For older adults, particularly those who are frail and with limited capacity to recover, any illness can lead to long-term functional decline. People like me, working in hospitals with older adults, have worried about this for a long time.

At the same time, for someone who has had a mild illness, I would worry about getting dementia after COVID-19 no more than if they'd had a cold.

If you are worried about COVID-19 increasing your risk of dementia, I have a simple solution: vaccination. The vaccines are excellent at preventing severe disease, and if you avoid severe disease, you are protecting your brain.

Can we control inflammation?

There are medications that are used to control serious autoimmune diseases, such as lupus or inflammatory bowel disease. These medications dramatically suppress the immune system, but come with significant risks, including increasing the risk of infection. Aging, especially reaching very old age, is also invariably associated with a decline in specific immunity and less control of inflammation, since the damage to cells that comes with aging can mean that the immune system is more active, even when there isn't a new threat.

It is also key to remember that the entire point of the immune system is to be interconnected to create a whole-body response. The immune system is in a constant delicate balance, saving our lives each and every day while perhaps doing a little damage along the way.

As you'll see over the following pages, inflammation is also influenced by almost everything in life, including stress, exercise, sleep, and even the microbes in our gut.

Does dementia begin in the gut?

James came to see me with his son Martin. I started asking James and Martin about James's Parkinson's disease. I asked about sleep, blood pressure problems, falls, and medication side effects. Initially, James and Martin denied hallucinations when I asked about them, but when I specifically asked whether he ever saw little ants or insects, Martin suddenly realized that the little ants his dad was always squashing with his walking stick were actually hallucinations.

The key features of Parkinson's disease are a stooped shuffling walk, a blank, expressionless face, a "pill rolling" tremor of the index finger and thumb, and freezing in movement. These fall under the broad category of movement disorders. By the time someone has had the disease for twenty years or more, they will almost all have some cognitive dysfunction.

Somewhere between 50 and 80 percent of all people with Parkinson's disease have constipation, which can start decades before the motor symptoms. Constipation in Parkinson's disease is caused by slow transit—the intestines don't move the food through the gut as fast as they should. Indeed, in a study of men who were followed for six years and were classified by the number of bowel movements they had per day, those who had a bowel movement three times a week or less were almost five times as likely to be diagnosed with Parkinson's disease compared to those who had a bowel movement once a day.

One day, we may be able to make an early diagnosis of Parkinson's disease by a gastroscopy. Studies on animals and humans have identified that clumps of an abnormal protein called "alpha-synuclein" can be found in the gut, and these are associated with alpha-synuclein clumps in the brain. It may be that these clumps can travel directly up the vagus nerve, which connects our brains to our other organs, including the lungs, heart, and intestines. Alpha-synuclein deposits are also associated with increased gut permeability, which could explain why people with Parkinson's disease are more likely to have bacteria that have penetrated the mucosal lining of the gut, although it could also be the other way around. Some people with Parkinson's seem to have a predominance of species in their "microbial garden" that produce less of the beneficial short-chain fatty acids (SCFAs), which are a source of energy for the lining of the intestine and help with gut health.

It's an incredible thought that one day we could make an early diagnosis of Parkinson's disease by a gut biopsy, particularly if it leads to early treatments for this difficult to treat, progressive condition.

Parkinson's disease is also only one neurological condition with links to the gut. There are other types of dementia that you can actually get from food that travels through the gut. More on that shortly.

What is the gut?

Our digestive system is built on an essential conflict. Its purpose is to absorb the nutrients and water we need to survive, while preventing the trillions of microbes present in our digestive tract from invading our bodies. It's not an easy task.

Our gut, more formally known as our digestive tract, extends from our mouth to our anus. It is basically one long tube, with different parts having different structures and functions. The food we eat passes through all these parts so we can extract nutrients from it.

The digestive tract is a really great place for microbes to live. It's at a constant temperature, there's a constant level of moisture, and there is a steady and reliable source of food coming by; it's no wonder that many microbes have become perfectly adapted to life in the gut.

While every section of the gut has its own microbial flora, the most heavily populated area is our large intestine, which is the final 1.5 meters starting in the right lower abdomen, traveling up to the liver, across to the spleen, then down to the rectum and anus. Not that long ago, we thought that the only role of the large intestine was to absorb water, but now we know that the tiny microbes that live within it have a huge influence on health.

The specialist microbes living in the gut, known as "commensal bacteria," don't want to make us sick. It's not in their interest for their human host to die. They would much rather that we remain happy and healthy and feeding them fiber. Yet these microbes are not passive in making themselves a comfortable home. Over the course of evolution, they have evolved ways and means to influence their human hosts. In turn, we have evolved ways and means to keep them in check. A breakdown of this delicate balance has been implicated in many chronic diseases, including dementia.

A gut feeling

Have you ever had a sinking feeling in your gut? Perhaps butterflies in your stomach? Felt nauseous with anxiety?

So many of the phrases we use to describe a strong feeling refer to feelings within our bodies. The emotions derived from our brain are experienced as something physical. The thing is, this relationship between the brain and gut is actually bidirectional. Some of our thoughts, behaviors, and emotions actually start in the depths of our intestines.

The gut–brain axis is the link between our brain and our intestinal environment; it's a link between our thoughts, behaviors, and feelings. While we may feel like our brains are in charge of our bodies, our thoughts, feelings, and behaviors are strongly influenced by our gut, which has its own nervous system. While our brains have 100 billion neurons, our gut has 500 million neurons—around the same number as the brain of a cat.

Our gut isn't just doing the work of extracting energy from food: It is also a sensory organ that sends signals back to the brain via both the vagus nerve and by hormones. We actually have a large nervous system in our gut, which is important for coordinating digestion, including propelling food through the digestive tract in an orderly manner while releasing the right digestive enzymes at the right time. Just as we think of our skin as a sensory organ, our gut is also a sensory organ.

While our brains do send signals to the gut, there is actually a lot more information traveling the other way. The vagus nerve travels from the base of the brain and wanders through the body to innervate our organs. In the gut, 90 percent of this nerve is actually transmitting information back to the brain. There is also evidence that abnormal proteins can travel to the brain this way. This could be one of the ways that diseases start in the brain.

The other way our gut communicates with the brain is via hormones—chemical signals that travel via the blood. When our stomach is empty, it releases a hormone called "ghrelin" into the blood (I always remembered this as the "growly" tummy hormone). When the stomach is stretched, it releases leptin, which helps us feel full.

Our gut bacteria also play a role in mood regulation by making neurotransmitters, such as serotonin and gamma-aminobutyric acid (GABA). Serotonin seems to have important effects on mood. One of the most commonly prescribed types of antidepressants are selective serotonin reuptake inhibitors (SSRIs).

Serotonin is a great example of the way our body can repurpose different chemicals at the cellular level to work on many different cell types. Receptors for serotonin are present on gut cells, nerve cells, and even platelets, which are small cell fragments that help our blood to clot. Serotonin also helps to regulate inflammation.

Gut bacteria don't produce serotonin for our benefit: they produce serotonin to regulate their own environment, and in doing so can impact their human hosts.

When our microbes have a lovely meal of fiber, they produce bioactive metabolites called "short-chain fatty acids." SCFAs provide around 10 percent of a person's daily calories and they are a particularly important source of nutrition for gut enterocytes (intestinal absorptive cells). These also act as cell signalers and help us to feel full after a meal (think about that—you're not full until your microbes say you are full!). These SCFAs may also influence our moods. One of these, butyrate, has been identified as particularly important in depression. Butyrate supplements may one day be a treatment for depression.

All of this means that the brains in our head are in a constant bidirectional conversation with the brains in our gut, and maintaining that balance is critical to our health.

How do we absorb nutrients and keep bacteria out?

Most nutrients are absorbed in the small intestine. The inside surface of the small intestine is covered in folds to increase the available area for absorption. The layer of cells defining the inside and outside of the intestines is only one cell thick. A key role of these "epithelial cells" is maintaining the integrity of the gut barrier, and they are tightly joined together to prevent bacteria passing through. The cells have a hard life as they are being pummeled by food all day, so they turn over every few days.

Underneath the epithelial cells on the inside of the gut is a thin layer of connective tissue. Between the microbes in the hollow tube of the gut and the epithelial cells is a layer of mucus. This slimy layer is critical in shielding the inside of the gut from bacterial products.

Since the gut is the frontier of our bodies, a staggering 70 percent of the body's immune system resides there. The intestinal epithelial cells also form part of this immune system. They are capable of ingesting bacteria and are in regular communication with other immune cells in the gut, which play a role in regulating the immune response to bacterial products.

The cells lining the inside of the gut also respond to chemical immune signals, cytokines, which control their activity, and when there are higher levels of inflammatory signals, the gut lining becomes more permeable to allow more immune cells to migrate to the gut. This also exposes more bacterial products to the blood stream. Ideally, we want this inflammation and permeability to turn on and off quickly, but sometimes it can become dysregulated, and a low level of inflammation remains.

Our immune cells also need to know the difference between the "good" gut bacteria that they should tolerate and the "bad" bacteria that are causing a problem, like telling the difference between a friend or foe. If there is a disruption to the recognition of the helpful bacteria, and they start to be treated like enemies, this actually gives the enemies an advantage and they start to take over.

Having a compromised intestinal barrier is associated with many chronic diseases, such as diabetes and heart disease, as well as autoimmune diseases like rheumatoid arthritis. One of the biggest questions in science at the moment is whether this is the cause or consequence of systemic inflammation.

It is highly plausible that having an increased level of gut permeability causes disease because it means that there is an increased exposure to bacterial toxins. This can activate the systemic inflammation, which is linked to so many chronic diseases.

When there are higher levels of systemic inflammation, the blood–brain barrier becomes more permeable, and the microglia, the immune cells of the brain, become active.

What is the link between the gut microbiome and dementia?

The types of microbes we have in our gut may play an important role in the development of dementia.

In a study that looked at a group of 128 patients in Japan who attended a clinic for memory assessment, on average, people who were diagnosed with dementia had different ratios of bacterial species from those without. People who were diagnosed with dementia were less likely to have *bacteroides* species and more *firmicutes*. This also corresponded to an increased likelihood of subclinical brain infarcts, or small areas of dead tissue, as seen on an MRI.

The same research group then looked at fecal metabolites and found more key differences. People with a higher level of ammonia, which is a neurotoxin, in their feces were more likely to have dementia.

The short-chain fatty acids that our gut bacteria produce may also help to protect us against developing dementia. These can act to interfere with the production of amyloid-beta in our gut. They also influence the behavior of microglia, the immune cells in the brain. In trials using mouse models of dementia, it was seen that the presence of the SCFA butyrate actually improved cognition and decreased the damage that is characteristic of mouse Alzheimer's. While "mouseheimer's" is not the same as Alzheimer's, eating lots of fiber still seems like a good idea.

Gut permeability, cerebrovascular disease, and Type 2 diabetes

Some researchers have worked out ways to measure gut permeability in humans, by feeding the research subjects certain markers and then measuring how much appears in the blood and feces. These studies have enabled some remarkable findings, namely that the leakier the gut, the more likely it is that someone will experience metabolic endotoxemia. This occurs because the immune system is extremely sensitive to common proteins found on the outside of bacterial cells, and so inflammation rapidly increases.

How does this affect the brain? We know that increased permeability means increased exposure to bacterial products, which activates our immune system. When our immune system is active, our blood–brain barrier, which regulates brain exposure to the rest of the body, becomes a little more open. This then influences how active the microglia are and can make them less effective at turning off. This, in turn, sets up chronic inflammation in the brain and is the reason why many scientists believe that protecting gut integrity is key to preventing dementia.

The other link between intestinal permeability and dementia is blood vessel health. Increased inflammation, for any reason, can lead to damage to the blood vessels that are critical to brain health.

The most obvious example of the deleterious consequences of gut permeability is inflammatory bowel diseases, such as Crohn's disease and ulcerative colitis. In Crohn's disease, the inflammation can occur anywhere along the digestive tract. In ulcerative colitis, only the large intestine is affected. These diseases occur when there is a breakdown of the gut barrier and exposure to immune cells triggers uncontrolled inflammation. People can develop bloody diarrhea, weight loss, malnutrition, and even holes in the intestines that can sometimes go all the way to the skin or into other organs, such as the bladder. When a gastroenterologist performs a colonoscopy, they will often see bleeding ulcers. People with these conditions will often need powerful immune-suppressing medication.

One study found that people with inflammatory bowel disease had a higher incidence of dementia, at 5.5 percent versus 1.4 percent among control subjects. They are also diagnosed with dementia around seven years earlier. This is another important clue to understanding dementia.

It's highly plausible that for many types of neurodegenerative conditions, the gut seems to play a key role by regulating systemic inflammation as well as the direct effects of the microbes on the function of our nervous system.

To me, this is one of the most exciting areas of science because of the potential for treatments, particularly with chemicals like butyrate, which has already shown promise in small trials of treatment for depression. It is also exciting because there is an obviously actionable message for the here and now: eat your veggies!

Edible dementia

From 1996, there was a ban on British beef in Australia. Bovine spongiform encephalopathy (BSE), also known as "mad cow disease," is a disease caused by prions. Prions are a very weird concept to understand—they are abnormally folded proteins that cause other proteins to become abnormally folded, and thus spread through the nervous system. While prion diseases can arise spontaneously, you can also "catch" them by ingesting meat from infected animals. In humans, these prions cause a rapidly progressive dementia called Creutzfeldt-Jakob disease (CJD). This is a relentless and awful form of dementia, and few people live more than a year after diagnosis. The earliest symptoms are usually psychiatric, including anxiety, depression, and sometimes paranoia. The British beef ban arose because there was an outbreak of CJD related to infected beef. This occurred because farmers were feeding their cows with meal that contained ground-up animal products, so the cows were eating other cows with BSE.

Humans can also catch a prion form of dementia from eating other humans. In the highlands of Papua New Guinea, there is a disease called "kuru." It comes on differently than CJD, with the early symptoms being difficulty walking and tremors. Within a year, victims can no longer get off the floor. The disease primarily affects women and young children. In these villages, it was customary to consume the dead as an act of love and grief. The body was primarily consumed by women, who would give pieces to their children. Once researchers made the link between consuming bodies and kuru, the practice stopped and the epidemic ended.

Prions break a lot of our scientific rules about infectious agents: they don't have DNA; however, they are still contagious. While it's not completely clear how they move from the gut to the brain, eating infected meat is a clear pathway to infection.

What these conditions do show definitively is that it is possible to get a brain disease from something in the gut. Some post-mortem studies have shown evidence of prions in the vagus nerve, so that may be a pathway.

Does stress cause dementia?

Stress

Stress is an unavoidable part of life. It is often necessary in making great achievements, but it can also be unrelenting and have measurable negative impacts on memory and thinking. Stress is also linked with depression and anxiety. To make this more confusing, depression and anxiety can also impair cognitive function, and so can mimic dementia. I know when my brain is getting overloaded, I have trouble remembering everything I need to do. I have trouble sleeping, my memory gets a little foggy, it's harder to focus, and I can get a little grumpy (apologies to my family!).

While a little stress can be good for brain function, like making us extra alert for an exam, when stress is constant and accompanied by a feeling of being out of control it is harmful.

Having a stress response can enhance memory and be important for our survival: we want to remember the danger. I don't remember all the minutiae of the hundreds of times I have taken my children to the park, but I vividly remember the time I lost my two-year-old because he decided to walk himself home. The minutes he was lost felt like an eternity until I found him with a kind stranger. Even writing this, I feel a small surge of dread at the thought of something bad happening to my child.

Remembering threatening events can be very useful. If you were a hunter-gatherer and there was a particular cave where once you saw a lion, that sharp fear-memory would help you avoid ever going near there again. We can gain another advantage by anticipating a threat before it happens. When we, or indeed any animal, see, smell, or hear something that is a threat to our survival, our stress system kicks into action. This critical head-start might mean the difference between surviving an attack or not. It's just that in modern life, the "threats" are things like a tight work deadline, not the need to escape a rival with a spear.

When we detect a threat, like seeing something scary, our sympathetic nervous system activates. Our hearts beat faster, our breathing becomes more rapid, our pupils dilate, and we sweat. It happens in a second. Stress also activates a gland on top of the kidney called the "adrenal medulla" and releases mineralocorticoid.

The other part of this response is the hypothalamic-pituitary-adrenal response. The hypothalamus and pituitary gland are in the brain. The hypothalamus tells the pituitary to release a hormone into the blood, which then tells the adrenal glands, which sit on top of the kidneys, to release glucocorticoid. Mineralocorticoid and glucocorticoid are both types of stress hormones that help prepare the body for a physical threat. The stress hormones travel through the bloodstream, so they take minutes, not seconds, to work, but they also last longer. The main glucocorticoid is cortisol. It acts on receptors in various organs to raise blood pressure, increase clotting, and raise blood glucose, which is very helpful if you are about to get injured and lose blood but not so helpful when you are stuck in traffic and running late.

These hormones also get into your brain and have different effects. Mineralocorticoid activates receptors in the amygdala and hippocampus and makes neurons in these regions more excitable, thereby making us alert and priming our memories. Cortisol also affects which genes are switched on, which impacts cellular activity. This takes around forty to sixty minutes to take effect but eventually slows down neural excitability to help the brain return to normal. As mentioned, a consequence of the stress response is that the memory is sharpened. Paradoxically, chronic stress may have a negative impact on our memory and thinking because over time, it seems, the brain becomes insensitive to this stress response.

With these responses, our bodies and brains are ready for "fight or flight." We are alert, thinking sharply, and ready to run or face attack. The problem is that in modern life, our threats are generally not wild animals but psychological in nature.

The impact of excess glucocorticoid

An extreme example of excess cortisol over a long period of time occurs in Cushing's syndrome. Cushing's *disease* is when a brain tumor signals to the adrenal glands to make too much cortisol. Cushing's *syndrome* is when this overproduction occurs due to another cause, such as receiving too much prednisolone, a cortisol commonly prescribed for autoimmune diseases such as inflammatory arthritis. Whatever the cause of the excess cortisol, the effect on the body is essentially the same. Common side effects are weight gain around the abdomen along with a loss of muscle mass in the arms and legs. Excess cortisol also suppresses the immune system (which is why synthetic forms of this are used for autoimmune diseases) and leads to the skin becoming thin and delicate. It also affects the brain, sometimes leading to depression, irritability, and occasionally even psychosis. Some people also develop cognitive impairment.

Chronic exposure to glucocorticoid makes neurons in the hippocampus less able to connect with one another. In an experiment with rats, those given daily injections of cortisol had a reduced number of hippocampal cells. They also had fewer cortisol receptors on their brain cells, likely a mechanism to try to minimize the metabolic load of constant activity. In mice, glucocorticoids also downregulate the expression of brain-derived neurotrophic factor, which is involved in learning by promoting connections between neurons. This may be one of the ways excess stress impacts learning.

When looking at neurons, mice and rats are far easier to study than humans. The poor animals get "sacrificed," to use the sanitized laboratory word for "killed," so that their brains can be studied. There is a high degree of similarity between the brains of humans and the brains of rats, and for a really important hormone pathway, such as for stress hormones, it is reasonable to think there are similar effects.

One of the key differences between the lab situation and real life is that many of the experiments on lab rats involves injecting them for months with glucocorticoids, which is obviously not the same as a human with a stressful life. We also can't ethically put humans under a huge amount of stress for a long time just to see what happens to their memories. We can only study the effects of stress by looking at people who have gone through difficult experiences.

Post-traumatic stress disorder (PTSD)

PTSD occurs after someone experiences an event that threatens their life or the life of someone else. The trauma can be a physical or sexual assault, a car crash, medical illness, living through war or disaster, or witnessing traumatic events, such as with police work. Some people experience multiple traumatic events. People with PTSD have a heightened state of arousal and can suffer nightmares, flashbacks, and severe anxiety. They might avoid things that trigger distressing memories, including people or places associated with the event. People can also feel numb, disconnected, and unable to find joy. Since mental health resources are so stretched, many people with PTSD don't get adequate treatment. As a consequence, some of them abuse alcohol or other drugs to try to cope with their symptoms. People who have PTSD have decreased speed of thinking, working memory, and attention. Imagine frequent and unpredictable memory incursions of the worst thing that ever happened to you. It's an awful thing to live with.

People with PTSD are around twice as likely to be diagnosed with dementia as those without. When researchers have tried to understand why, with MRI and neuropsychological testing, they have seen evidence of accelerated brain aging, including a decrease in the size of the hippocampus in PTSD sufferers. It is possible that the constant activation of stress systems causes metabolic stress, which ultimately damages neurons.

Stress, depression, and dementia

When a patient comes to see me with memory problems, especially if they are self-reported, one of the questions I ask myself is whether this is depression or dementia.

There is a lot of crossover in the early symptoms of dementia and the early symptoms of depression. One of the earliest symptoms of dementia is apathy, a loss of drive and motivation to do things, including previously enjoyable activities. This can look a lot like depression, and it means it is very difficult to differentiate between the two later in life.

Where we particularly need to look is at midlife depression and dementia risk. In a study of 13,535 people in the US, people with depression between the ages of forty and fifty-five were around 20 percent more likely to be diagnosed with dementia in follow-up decades later. Even with a break of forty years between depressive symptoms and dementia diagnosis, we still can't be completely sure that the depressive symptoms represent early signs of dementia and not a recurrence of depression.

Depression is a very complex illness. It is the result of social, psychological, and biological factors. Many of these are outside someone's control, like being made unemployed or having insecure housing; others are less so—for example getting exercise, good nutrition, and adequate sleep. For some people, depression appears to be part of a low-level inflammatory response related to lifestyle factors and the gut microbiome.

The hippocampus is highly sensitive to stress, and many animal studies have shown that it undergoes structural changes with stress. Since depression can also be brought on by severe stress, it is not surprising that moderate to severe depression is associated with a decrease in the size of the hippocampus when viewed on MRI. This is also associated with poorer memory function.

Helen

Helen lay awake, sweating, thoughts racing. She checked her bedside clock: it was 4 a.m., and all she could think about was how she was going to get her daughter to her dance dress rehearsal and get her mother to the doctor. The dress rehearsal also meant that she needed to get going with the sewing for the costume. So many sequins. What if her mother's bleeding was cancer? Her husband snored gently beside her, and she felt a flush of rage that he could sleep when she couldn't. She knew that was stupid and felt guilty, then remembered that his brother and his wife were coming for dinner on the weekend; what diet was she on now? She felt down to her pajamas, drenched with sweat from her hot flush; she felt her soft tummy, thinking she really needed to get to the gym as her clothes would stop fitting soon. Helen gave up on sleep and got up to make a start on folding the washing.

Helen was exhausted from not sleeping, and even during the day, anxious thoughts flew around her mind, gripping her, making her feel edgy, irritated. Wine took the edge off but made her sleep even worse. Her doctor gave her a new type of pill: Valium, he told her, would help and wasn't addictive.

I met Helen after she had been on diazepam for decades. When it was first prescribed, doctors didn't know it was addictive. I meet a lot of people who have been on benzodiazepines for decades and now struggle to stop taking them. The drivers for anxiety are complex, but psychological techniques to overcome it can help. The problem is, once someone has well-established dementia, it can be hard or impossible to learn these techniques, and so weaning off the benzodiazepines becomes very difficult.

Anxiety and dementia

Generalized anxiety disorder is defined as persistent and excessive worrying. People with anxiety have distressing thoughts that get stuck on a loop. It is often associated with poor sleep and physical symptoms like fatigue. Older adults with anxiety but without dementia have reduced verbal memory, language, and executive functions.

Multiple studies have shown that anxiety in midlife is a risk factor for dementia in later life. This association may be even stronger than for depression. The incredibly difficult issue in all this is to pick apart when anxiety and depression are part of mental illness and when they are the first symptoms of dementia. Many studies try to account for this by following people over a long time or looking at episodes of depression or anxiety that predate the diagnosis of dementia by around ten years. Nevertheless it is impossible to be sure.

In reading the research, from animal studies to human population cohorts, I can't help wondering whether midlife depression is simply an earlier manifestation of the same process that is causing dementia. As mentioned, certain structures in the brain, particularly the hippocampus, are incredibly sensitive to things like stress. The hippocampus is such an active part of the brain, so does this make it more vulnerable to the hormonal and neurological impacts of chronic stress?

Depression, anxiety, and PTSD undoubtedly have an adverse impact on our brain function. Chronic exposure to glucocorticoids and the metabolic impact of stress on our neurons is not good for our ability to think clearly. Whether or not it definitively causes dementia, which I think is highly likely, it is also really unpleasant. Mental health conditions can have a huge impact on people's lives. Thankfully, they are also treatable if you have access to people who can help. I recommend starting with your doctor.

Depression is an inflammatory illness

A highly plausible link between depression and dementia is inflammation. When you are sick, you feel lethargic, have trouble concentrating, and just want to stay in bed. It is very hard to find the energy to do the things necessary to get through the day. This is very similar to depression. It is actually possible to induce depression with medications that stimulate inflammation. Prior to the development of new, more effective drugs, part of the treatment for hepatitis C was injected interferon, a potent stimulator of the immune system. One of the problems with this treatment was that a substantial number of people—15 to 40 percent—couldn't tolerate it because it caused major depression.

As well as getting the body ready for physical exertion, stress activates the immune system. This makes sense from an evolutionary perspective, because if you are in a fight you might be injured and a rapid immune response will help stop infection and aid healing. Higher levels of inflammation also make us very tired, which may be another mechanism to force us to conserve energy for healing.

It may be that some people, particularly those with trauma in their early life, have a stronger inflammatory response to stress than the general population. Some of the most compelling evidence for this comes from Dunedin, where 1,037 people have been followed since infancy with repeated assessments. At the age of thirty two, people with higher levels of childhood maltreatment had higher levels of inflammatory biomarkers on blood tests.

Social isolation and dementia

In a study of 2,038 people who were followed for ten years, the dementia risk was tripled for people who were otherwise at low risk if they reported that they were lonely. Loneliness is something that is subjective. Some people enjoy their own company; some people live with others and still feel lonely (this is a big problem in assisted living).

A few years ago, there was a study published that got a lot of attention in the media because it reported that isolation was as bad for you as smoking, and that it was a risk factor for early death. Social isolation is a form of psychological stress, which activates our stress response systems as described earlier.

Social isolation also means a lost opportunity for cognitive challenge.

This will be covered more in upcoming pages. In the meantime, think about being at a dinner party when a challenging topic comes up. You need to pull ideas and facts from your memory while responding to someone else's opinion. You may dislike their opinion intensely, but you also need to use your skill in emotional regulation not to say something inflammatory. It is a great stretch for the brain. Staying home all day with your own thoughts means one less way to exercise your brain.

Peter

Peter still remembers the last time he saw his mother. She had tried so hard to be cheery, and so he had done the same, but as he stood in the doorway of the group home, looking back at her, the tears started streaming down her face. His mom had told him it would only be for a little while, that she'd get a job and a nice home and he wouldn't be hungry anymore. At the group home, they were told that they were rubbish and that their parents didn't want them. Peter thought this must be true; otherwise, why would his mom have sent him away?

At the home, Peter never knew when he would be beaten, and he could never relax because the slightest thing was enough for one of the adults to get their cane. At first, Mr. Frost seemed different. He took Peter to his office and actually spoke to him like he mattered. But then it got worse. The first time Mr. Frost raped him, he tried to fight it. Afterward, he learned to pretend he was floating on the ceiling until it was over.

When Peter was fourteen, he left school and got a job on the docks. His boss was kind and told him he could live with him as long as he started night school. Peter particularly loved math, and he was good at it. Somehow, he managed to do well enough to finish high school and get a scholarship to the university. Life went well for Peter after this. He worked as an engineer, married, and became a loving father, but when he retired his early life kept coming back. He couldn't sleep, his thoughts raced, and he couldn't bear to go out. He forgot things, but not his trauma. He lost interest in seeing friends and even family.

The memories he had tried to suppress were branded on his brain. He became stuck in these pathways and in the intense distress of remembering. He couldn't concentrate, and his memory started to falter.

When Peter saw his doctor, he was clearly distressed, and his doctor diagnosed PTSD. As Peter also had memory problems, his doctor referred him to a psychiatrist for older age patients. While Peter did have cognitive deficits on testing, his psychiatrist held off on giving him a diagnosis of dementia until Peter's PTSD was treated.

Mental health is health

Even now, there is an urgent need to improve availability and access to treatments for mental health conditions. In the past, this was even worse. I see a lot of older adults who have had mental health conditions their whole lives and who have had no or inadequate treatment.

I regularly see people who have been incredibly resilient after childhood trauma, had good jobs, and created loving families. A lot of older adults have been through major stressors, like the loss of a child, being a refugee, or having an abusive parent, and have still gone on to be very functional adults.

It is in older age, when perhaps thinking is a little more rigid or there is some cognitive slowing, that these problems can come back and be harder to deal with. Once someone has been diagnosed with dementia, anxiety can be very hard to manage because it can be harder to learn psychological strategies to manage symptoms.

While it is hard to prove that the incessant hypervigilant loops of thought that occur in a condition like anxiety cause dementia, or that the feeling of mental slowness in depression can change thought processes forever, untreated mental health conditions contribute significantly to poor health through life. Getting treatment may decrease your risk of dementia, but even more, it will improve quality of life.

Of course, it is easy to write these words, but it is much harder to address why it is so difficult for people to get the help they need for mental health conditions. And while psychiatric medications can be highly effective, they don't make up for just how hard it is to get ongoing psychological help for mental health conditions. It is easy for a doctor to prescribe a medication, but seeing a psychiatrist and psychologist can be expensive, if there is even one available to see. The difficulty is only increased for people in rural areas.

Living a human life means there will be stresses and challenges, and often the best things in life come from this. For instance, having children certainly makes life more hectic, but raising my children is one of the best parts of my life. Overcoming difficulties can even lead to post-traumatic growth. How well people can cope with this is often due to the supports they have, both in terms of family and friends but also in terms of community and formal resources.

The thought I want to leave you with on this topic is that stress and challenges are not evenly distributed between people. I am very often struck by how very unfair life can be. Not just by what some people experience in their lives, but also by the fact that they don't necessarily have the resources available to enhance their lives with treatment. One of the myths of health is that we are all on an equal footing. The reality is, people with more money have less stress and more ability to get treatment. This is why health, particularly a life-course condition like dementia, needs to be looked at through a social lens. We will do this later in the book.

Is there medication to treat dementia?

It's really satisfying, for myself and my patients, when someone has a symptom or a disease and I can just prescribe a pill to make it all go away. I cannot tell you how much I wish I had a pill I could prescribe for dementia. Right now, we don't have any medications that stop the progression of any of the diseases. This is the story of why it is so hard to develop a treatment for something so common.

The long game

Like most age-related diseases, including cardiovascular disease, arthritis, and diabetes, the actual disease process in dementia starts decades before the symptoms. Someone doesn't wake up one day and suddenly have dementia; it is a continuous process. This creates a very serious problem in recruiting people for clinical trials.

Phase one trials are the first time humans are given the drug. The people recruited for phase one trials don't need to have the medical condition being studied. The purpose of phase one trials is to see whether humans can tolerate the drug without side effects and at what dose, based on a best guess from animal studies. Phase two trials are done to see if it looks like the drug might work. A group of people with the disease of interest are given the drugs and observations are made as to whether it looks like it is working or not. In phase three drug trials, a group of people with the disease are randomly assigned to have the treatment or a placebo, and results are collated. This is the last stage before a drug can be approved for the public—assuming it shows that it is an effective treatment. There are usually over a thousand people involved in this stage of a drug trial, although this varies widely. After a drug has been approved, there is ongoing monitoring to look for very rare side effects.

For patients with cancer, phase one and two trials usually recruit people with advanced cancer who have a disease that has progressed through conventional treatments. Because of their perilous situation, participants will take the risk of an adverse drug reaction; they have little to lose.

Recruiting the right patients for dementia trials is far more difficult. By the time someone has advanced dementia, their brains have suffered irreversible damage. In addition, as a general rule, someone with advanced dementia lacks capacity to consent to a drug trial, which presents an ethical issue. The goal in recruiting people for phase three trials of dementia drugs is to find those who are still early in the disease process, or even better, those who have yet to show any symptoms.

Most drug trials have focused on people with mild disease or mild cognitive impairment. The challenge in this is that not everyone with mild cognitive impairment will actually get dementia. It would be ideal to recruit people who are at risk of getting dementia but don't have it yet, but we don't have accurate ways to predict who will get dementia. Even for people with mild cognitive impairment, a substantial proportion will improve over time. While it would be possible to take a group of people in their fifties and randomize them to trial a drug or placebo, it would take decades to get a meaningful clinical result, and the number of people in the trial would be huge. I think it would be a very hard sell to get people to participate.

Some drug trials have recruited people who carry a gene that almost guarantees they will get younger onset dementia. Unfortunately, even trials in this group have not been effective, and even if a drug was effective in this group, this doesn't automatically mean that it will be effective in spontaneous Alzheimer's disease.

When I look at the criteria for patients to be enrolled in the trial of aducanumab, one of the most hyped dementia drugs of recent years, which I discuss below, I see that anyone with significant cerebrovascular disease wasn't eligible. Since we know that patients in their eighties and beyond almost all have mixed pathology, including vascular disease and Alzheimer's, basically none of my patients would have been eligible to be part of the trial. Indeed, the average age of people in the trial was seventy.

One of the other challenges in designing trials for dementia is choosing an outcome measure. We want a drug that will prevent dementia, or at least slow the decline. It may seem simple to just monitor to see if participants don't get dementia, but this is incredibly complex. It is challenging to use the right cognitive test, one that will have the right sensitivity and specificity to detect a meaningful change that would eventually translate to at least delaying disability and death.

Dementia is also not just about the score on a test. What really matters is how the person with dementia is doing in everyday life. This is why many studies also use subjective measures, which means clinical judgment based on assessment of the person with dementia and input from someone who knows them well. Because of this, and reliance on the judgment of the researchers, it is important that trials are blinded, which means that the participants and researchers do not know if they are on the active drug or the placebo.

The ideal treatment for dementia is one that stops the disease in its tracks before people get symptoms, but how do we choose an outcome measure for people with no symptoms? One that has been used is whether a drug can clear amyloid. This brings us to a huge recent controversy in the quest for a treatment for Alzheimer's: the drug aducanumab, which was recently approved in the United States.

The aducanumab story

"Doctor, isn't there something else we can try?"

My patient's husband is begging me for another option. He is watching his wife's mind fade away. He wants her back; he is so lonely. None of the available medications have worked to improve her symptoms of dementia. I have no other treatment to offer. It is heartbreaking.

Yet in 2021 when the US Food and Drug Administration (FDA) announced that they had approved the first new treatment for Alzheimer's disease since 2003, I was shocked. Indeed, three members of the advisory board who had recommended the FDA should not approve this drug actually resigned in protest.

This may seem like a surprising reaction for someone who treats Alzheimer's disease. Haven't we all been waiting for a treatment to stop the relentless, devastating process? Why is this so controversial?

Aducanumab is given by intravenous infusion every month with gradual dose increases. Patients require regular monitoring with MRI because in clinical trials some people developed brain swelling and microhemorrhages. It was initially priced at $56,000 per patient per year, meaning that if one-third of the estimated 6 million people with Alzheimer's in the United States receives the new treatment, healthcare spending could swell by $112 billion annually. In 2020, Medicare spent $96 billion on pharmaceuticals, in total.

Aducanumab is a monoclonal antibody that can cross into the brain and amyloid plaques. Monoclonal antibodies are a type of drug that is engineered to activate the immune system. Aducanumab is very effective at clearing amyloid in the brain. In an early study of 165 people who took a placebo or varying drug doses, patients who could tolerate aducanumab developed negative amyloid PET scans. There was also a reduction in the rate of cognitive loss, although the study was not designed or powered to measure clinical outcomes.

The pharmaceutical company Biogen then went on to do two phase three trials. These were randomized controlled trials, where people were randomly assigned to a treatment or placebo group. People were eligible to be included if they were showing symptoms of early-stage dementia or had moderate dementia. There were strict exclusion criteria, including for people with cerebrovascular disease or stroke (so, excluding most older adults with dementia). Of the two phase three trials, ENGAGE, did not show any benefit in taking aducanumab. The other, called EMERGE, was initially stopped because of futility (an inability to reach the objectives of the trial). The Biogen share price plummeted. Biogen did not give up. (They initially called this push Project Phoenix, but after advice from lawyers they changed it to Project Onyx.) On an analysis with longer follow-up, there was a small benefit to people who received a high dose of aducanumab.

Based on this, in October 2020, Biogen announced they were going to apply for approval from the FDA.

An outside advisory committee, commissioned by the FDA, reviewed the evidence and were in almost unanimous agreement that the drug did not work, and that the high rate of brain swelling meant that it was dangerous.

Despite this, the drug was approved via the FDA's accelerated approval pathway. The accelerated approval pathway originally came about as the result of lobbying by AIDS activists in 1992. I'm sure we all remember the terrifying risk of HIV in the pre-antiretroviral era when people who were young and healthy would waste away and die. Since HIV was universally fatal, people with this condition were willing to take higher risks of harm from treatments because what was the point in being cautious if you were going to die anyway? People with HIV had no time to wait, and they, along with pharmaceutical companies, lobbied the FDA to speed up the process when a disease was fatal and there was no other treatment option. For AIDS, this was a huge success. While I have seen plenty of patients who are living with HIV as a chronic condition, stable on medications, I have never seen anyone with full-blown AIDS.

What the accelerated approval pathway does is allows for earlier approval of drugs that treat serious conditions and that fill an unmet medical need based on a surrogate endpoint. A surrogate endpoint is a marker, such as a laboratory measurement, radiographic image, physical sign, or other measure, that is thought to predict clinical benefit but is not itself a measure of clinical benefit. In the case of aducanumab, the surrogate endpoint was clearing amyloid from the brain. The accelerated approval still requires the drug company to prove it works. Biogen was given nine years to run this trial.

The FDA approved this drug because Alzheimer's is a devastating disease and there is a huge unmet need for treatment. Its decision was heavily influenced by patient perspectives, by people who felt they had no time to wait because of what they were already losing. It approved aducanumab because aducanumab reliably reduces amyloid plaques in the brain, and on the assumption that the amyloid hypothesis is correct, they reasoned it is "reasonably likely" to stop or reduce cognitive decline. There was also a consistent relationship between the reduction of amyloid and an improvement in a measure of cognitive function.

After the emergency-use approval, the trial results were published in a scientific journal, although not one of the most prestigious ones. While there was a statistically significant difference between people given a high dose of aducanumab, which means that the outcomes are unlikely to have occurred due to chance alone, there were problems with the results reported in the study. In addition, the difference between the outcomes of the control group and the placebo group was so small, it is unlikely to be noticeable in day-to-day life.

The FDA has an important role in making sure drugs are both safe and effective before they go to market. This means well-conducted, transparent clinical trials. This process takes years and costs hundreds of millions of dollars for the company developing a new drug. It also requires enough patients with the condition to make the process worthwhile.

The approval for aducanumab was staggeringly broad. Even though clinical trials had only been conducted in people with early-stage disease, it was initially approved for everyone at all stages of the disease, although this was subsequently revised to only those with mild cognitive impairment or early disease. There was no requirement for a diagnostic test, such as an amyloid PET scan, even though clinical diagnosis of different dementia types is far from perfect.

There are also serious safety concerns, with 35 percent of people in the trial receiving high-dose aducanumab showing amyloid-related imaging abnormalities (ARIA) and brain swelling compared to 2 percent in the placebo group. Of those in the high-dose group with brain swelling, around 40 percent had symptoms, and 1.5 percent had severe symptoms.

There were also concerns raised that there was an unusual degree of collaboration between the FDA and Biogen. It was reported on June 29, 2019, in STAT, a website reporting on pharmaceutical and medical news, that a top Biogen executive met with Billy Dunn, who is the agency's top regulator of Alzheimer's drugs, against FDA protocols, to enlist his support to approve aducanumab.

In a letter dated July 9, 2020, Dr. Janet Woodcock, the acting commissioner of the FDA, requested an independent review and assessment of interactions between representatives of Biogen and the FDA during the process leading to the decision to approve aducanumab, to determine whether any of those interactions were inconsistent with FDA policies and procedures. Biogen's share price again fell.

One of the conditions of the emergency-use authorization was that Biogen were given nine years to prove that aducanumab actually works. This meant they could potentially make billions of dollars in the interim. Even though the price of the drug was slashed a few months after release, due to interpretation of risks and benefits, very few doctors prescribed it.

The real nail in the coffin was when Medicare stated it would only cover aducanumab in the context of a clinical trial, the first time this had ever happened. Normally when the FDA approves a drug, Medicare agrees to pay for it.

Aducanumab was supposed to be a financial windfall for Biogen, but instead it has been a huge financial loss for the company, with sales amounting to just $1.3 million in 2021 and $2.8 million in the first three months of 2022. By mid-2022, Biogen had decided to stop marketing aducanumab altogether, basically giving up on it.

Some major figures have "retired" or moved on in the aftermath, and, while some of these people will walk away with the millions they have made, there are an estimated 1,000 other people who will lose their jobs.

"We just want more time"

Arthena was a fifty-six-year-old woman living with early-onset Alzheimer's, and a member of the board of the Alzheimer's association. She testified in front of the FDA in support of aducanumab. Arthena was diagnosed with dementia five years earlier, after she started having trouble with work. At the age of fifty-one she was told she only had five to ten years of life left, and that she would soon be dependent on others. While she was fully aware of the potential side effects, all she wanted was a chance to have more time with her family and more time to be independent. She wanted to be able to continue her advocacy work, as a black woman addressing health inequalities impacting people of color. She said that even if the drug only slowed the decline by months, she had nothing to lose.

Listening to Arthena is incredibly moving. She is a powerful speaker. I can feel her need for hope and can see why she wants access to a drug like aducanumab, despite the doubts that accompany it.

Consumer groups lobbied heavily for the approval of aducanumab, including the US's Alzheimer's Association, which drove a grassroots campaign called "More Time." featuring ordinary families and celebrities like Samuel L. Jackson. There were also paid advertisements from the Alzheimer's Association.

Here is the problem with the "grassroots" campaign: the US's Alzheimer's Association, which is a consumer advocate group, received $275,000 of funding from Biogen. They also receive funding from many other pharmaceutical companies.

I question whether a consumer advocate group can truly prioritize the interests of consumers when it is getting so much funding from pharmaceutical companies. And this is a shame, because it's people who need more time that deserve the most transparent advocacy.

What drugs are actually available for persons with dementia?

There are two classes of drugs that have been available for around two decades. Neither class is a cure, but in around a third of people they can somewhat improve symptoms such as memory loss.

I will be referring to all drugs by their proper names rather than their brand names. This is like using the word "tissues" rather than Kleenex.

Cholinesterase inhibitors

These drugs were introduced in 1997, and there are three different ones on the market: donepezil, galantamine, and rivastigmine. The cholinesterase inhibitors act by stopping the breakdown of acetylcholine, which is a neurotransmitter in the brain. In a review of ten randomized controlled trials, these drugs were seen to give small improvements in cognitive function over six months, as well as activities of daily living. Caregivers subjectively thought that people with dementia improved on these medications. Nevertheless, around 30 percent of people who start on one of these medications will stop because of side effects. The most common side effects are vomiting, nausea, diarrhea, and urinary incontinence. Less commonly, a more serious side effect is slowing of the heart rate, which can sometimes cause collapse.

Memantine

Memantine acts by blocking the receptor for the neurotransmitter glutamate. Glutamate is an excitatory neurotransmitter, and if it accumulates outside the neurons, it is bad for them. Memantine is effective in moderate to severe dementia. People generally don't get many side effects from it. Some studies have shown benefit from being on both memantine and a cholinesterase inhibitor, once dementia has progressed beyond mild. A one-month supply of memantine is around $40, and some people choose to pay the full amount to be on both.

The original drug trials for memantine and cholinesterase inhibitors only included people with a clinical diagnosis of Alzhiemer's disease, but since so many people have mixed pathology with Alzheimer's, vascular, and Lewy body dementia, it is reasonable to trial it with most people. It's also worth noting that the studies of these drugs were done before the development of specific diagnostic tools, such as PET scans, and so they likely included people with vascular dementia and Lewy body unintentionally.

Something to calm down

The use of sedating drugs is one of the most controversial in dementia care. Antipsychotic medications increase the risk of death for people with dementia, but they are still incredibly widely used. In a study that looked at 322,120 people living in nursing homes, almost 70,000 received an antipsychotic medication and over 98,000 received a benzodiazepine, which is a drug like Valium. Almost half of these people had not received these sedating medications before entering assisted living.

Antipsychotics do have an important role in managing distressing symptoms that can't be managed any other way. Some people "sundown" and become incredibly agitated and unhappy every evening. Others have unsettling hallucinations or delusions. Given that dementia is a terminal disease and many people experiencing the most distress are in the later stages of disease, these medications can reasonably be part of palliative care.

It is a complex problem, however. While there is a push to stop people prescribing antipsychotics in assisted living facilities, that needs to be in concert with addressing underlying issues in staff training and staff-to-resident ratios in these facilities, and in our system this leads to conflicts of interest. Many companies that run assisted living facilities in Australia are publicly listed, with an obligation to make profit for shareholders, and have no mandated staff-to-resident ratios. It is easier to manage people who are sedated and spend the day sleeping in a chair rather than up and about and needing engagement. This is not a criticism of the people who work in nursing homes, but of a system that profits from care of some of the most vulnerable people in society. I have more to say about this in a later chapter.

What is the future for dementia drugs?

The search for a treatment for Alzheimer's disease is far from over. In January 2022, there were 143 drugs in 172 clinical trials, with 31 in phase three trials, which is a trial designed to see if the drug is effective compared to a placebo, and usually the last stage before approval. Most of these trials were for disease-modifying drugs, the drugs that researchers hope will be a cure. Some drugs were "cognitive enhancers" and others were for neuropsychiatric symptoms. These drugs have a variety of different mechanisms. Some target amyloid, others tau; some are neuroprotective, and some target inflammation. Some of the drugs being studied have names like "NE3107," which means they are a very, very long way from the pharmacy shelves. I sincerely hope that one or more of these works to cure or at least slow the progression of dementia.

There is another line of research that may lead to drugs to delay the onset of dementia, which may come sooner, and this is repurposing of existing drugs. Metformin is an old and effective drug for type 2 diabetes. It acts to suppress the production of glucose in the liver and to increase sensitivity to glucose. It does this by acting on the mitochondria, which are the "organelles" inside the cells that break down glucose to make available energy.

One trial is recruiting people with mild cognitive impairment to see if the medication metformin can prevent dementia. If a trial like this shows benefit, and since metformin already has excellent long-term safety data, it could enter clinical practice for dementia in a few years.

The story is not finished

In 2023 lecanemab was approved by the FDA for treatment of early stage Alzheimer's disease. As I write this in mid-2024, it is likely that donanemab is going to be approved as well. In phase three clinical trials, both of these medications led to a moderate slowing of progression of cognitive decline in carefully selected patients.

Both lecanemab and donanemab have significant side effects, with brain swelling and microhemorrhages more common in the treatment arm than the placebo arm (lecanemab 30 percent versus 21 percent; donanemab 44 percent versus 9 percent). Overall, around 7 percent of people in the trial for lecanemab stopped treatment and for donanemab it was 8 percent. In the donanemab trial, out of 853 people, there were three deaths that were thought to be treatment-related.

These drugs are both given be infusion and require careful selection of patients as they must have a positive amyloid PET and to have only early stage disease. People on the medication also need to have regular MRIs to monitor for brain swelling and bleeds. People with two copies of the APOEE4 allele appear to be at a higher risk of brain bleeding.

These drugs are excellent at clearing amyloid from the brain, but they certainly don't stop disease progression. People in the trial who received the active drug still had a decline in their cognition. People with early stage dementia have a life expectancy of around eight to ten years, and the trials only ran for eighteen months, so there is still a big unanswered question about what will happen to people over a longer time period. It is also worth remembering that the average age in these trials was relatively young, at seventy-one in the lecanemab trial and seventy-three in the donanemab trial. People were also excluded from the lecanemab trial if they had MRI evidence of any other disease process on MRI. Since almost all adults aged over eighty will have a mixed picture, this would have knocked out most patients from trial eligibility. This is why it is always important to see how a drug works in a real-world setting, where patients are often quite different from trial participants.

I know some people are very optimistic that this is the start of a cure for Alzheimer's disease. While it would make me so happy if this turns out to be true, I am more circumspect. I am very much in the-wait-and-see-what-happens camp, but right now, I can say that, sadly, these drugs are not a cure.

How do we ethically distribute research dollars?

If the news on dementia drugs is not as optimistic as we would like, there is something we can take heart from. A study published in the medical journal *The Lancet* suggests that around a third of dementia cases can be prevented or delayed by adopting lifestyle changes. This is the subject of future chapters, but it is relevant to mention here in the context of public and private health efforts. As mentioned earlier, so many drugs have been trialed unsuccessfully and so much money has been spent to no avail that in 2018 drug company Pfizer announced it was pulling out of research into Alzheimer's and Parkinson's drugs.

So what if the money was spent in a different way? On ensuring that children get the best education, food, and lifestyle possible? On public health measures to make it easy for people in midlife to be active, to get enough sleep and social engagement, and to control cardiovascular risk factors like blood pressure? These efforts would probably deliver a more efficient use of funds than a drug treatment. The problem is these things can't be patented to make a profit.

QUESTION 11:

What is life like for a person living with dementia?

Then

The best moment was always just before she saw the beach. Legs and lungs burning as she ran up the sand dunes, pushing herself through the discomfort, feet sinking into the sand, her body saying it was too much but her mind pushing past the discomfort. She would reach the top and see the vast blue-gray ocean ahead of her, always there but always different. Until she reached the top she didn't know if it would be glassy or choppy, clear or swirling with sand. When it was hot, she would run down the steep dune—her legs sinking into the soft sand, the long grass whipping against her legs—and straight into the ocean. The shock of the cold was the most alive she ever felt.

Every day she ran, and every day it helped her to be calm and focused. It kept her happy. No matter what was planned for her

141

day, no matter how hard it got, she could always run along the dunes.

Now

In the nursing home, the corridors are endless. There is no wind, and everything looks the same. She walks and gets lost. She wants to go outside to run and see the beach, but when she tries to leave through the locked door, someone takes her arm and leads her back to the lounge. She doesn't know who these people are, the ones who speak in lilting baby tones. Once she did get out and she walked into traffic, narrowly avoiding being hit by a car. Her family was furious with the staff, so she has a sensor attached to her wrist that sets off a loud alarm every time she goes near the door. She feels a restless agitation and tries to draw on that activity that always used to help her—walking—to manage this stress. Instead, she gets labeled a "wanderer." Her walking is defined as a problem by everyone around her because no one has time to take her outside.

A person living with dementia

So far, I have written about neurons and synapses, chemical messengers, and microbes. I've described labels of disease and symptoms. The precise language of science is necessary for scientists and clinicians to communicate information among themselves. This language doesn't help me much when I sit with a patient with dementia. When I see someone who needs support to manage their life, a person who lives and loves, who has needs to be met and is doing their best to make sense of the world and feel safe, I try to soften my language to meet that need. Our existence and our actions are the result of chemical and electrical signals in the brain, but this does not make human experience any less incredible. Trying to understand other people, especially those who seem different from us, is one of the most important things we can do. You may know one person with dementia; you don't know every person with dementia. I've met many more than one, but I cannot capture a universal experience in just one person. Dementia is also progressive. The subjective experience of someone early in the process is likely to be very different from someone who is five to ten years after diagnosis.

If I try to draw a person, I will end up with a stick figure with only the most basic features. I fear this is the equivalent of the accounts I'm presenting in this book, as a cognitively able person writing about an ever-changing condition in the infinite variety of human life and experience, but I want to try to increase the understanding of advanced dementia because, for so many people, the first time they have experience with someone with advanced dementia, it is as their caregiver.

We all like to think that we can trust our memories, because what are we if not the version of self we hold in our heads? We make sense of the world based on what we know, and we are constantly drawing on things we have learned to be able to meet the next challenge. It's rare that anyone really asks the question "Who are you?" but it is always there in everyday life in the way we define ourselves, our jobs, our relationships to others, the music we enjoy, and the TV we want to watch.

As we grow and learn from childhood to adulthood, we learn to make sense of the world, we learn words, emotional regulation, the motor sequences of getting dressed or riding a bike. We learn how to control where we pass urine or feces, and we learn to care that this should be done in private and in a toilet.

People with dementia are exactly that: people

They are people who are trying to make sense of a world, trying to connect to with other humans, trying to solve problems in the face of decreased ability to remember, to integrate sensory input, to imagine, plan, and problem solve. They can forget the social rules, the emotional regulation, and how to define themselves.

While people with early or mild dementia, especially where language is spared, are able to describe much of their experience, it is the people in the later stage of the disease that I will focus on in the pages ahead. These are the people I meet every day at work, the people who, due to their cognitive disability, are less able to describe their own experiences. It is in this stage of dementia that it becomes harder to meet people's needs, since they can't always express them, and it can take special skill to make sure people have quality of life.

I'm waiting for Mom

Then

Samuel's favorite time of day was after dinner. His bath was done and his baby sister had gone to sleep, and this was when his mom would climb into bed to read to him. The days were so busy and rushed with school, football, friends, and chores, but in that moment, all was done, and Mom was all his. They would snuggle, and she would read to him stories from *The Faraway Tree* or *The Famous Five*. She always called him her "best boy." He would snuggle into her and close his eyes, feeling as safe, warm, and loved as could be.

Now

Samuel is worried; he doesn't know anyone around him. The place is strange; everyone has their faces covered so that he can't hear them. He can't work out what they are asking of him. He wants to feel safe; he wants that feeling of security. A woman comes to see him. She pulls her mask down and calls him "Dad." Her warm smile makes him feel better, but he is also uneasy. Why is this woman calling him Dad? He asks her when Mom is coming. Soon, she says, soon. She starts reading—it's from *The Faraway Tree*. She holds his hand. The voice is calm and loving, and he feels happy being there with Mom.

Most memories are like drawing on the skin with ink—they will wash away. A memory with strong emotion is like a tattoo, a permanent etching.

Our memories make us who we are, but people with dementia frequently lose the ability to make new memories. They also lose episodic memory; the memory of the story of life. People can experience a present that is far from the time they are actually in, such as the old man who is living the experience of a little boy who wants his mom. At least, wanting the love and security she made him feel.

Memory is inconsistent. Some people with dementia will only remember inconsistently that someone has died, even their life partner, leaving their family caught in a terrible bind when they ask for that person. Do they offer a comforting lie to the person or tell the truth, exposing fresh grief every time? At face value, it seems wrong and unethical to lie to someone with dementia. I see families who become so frustrated with the person when they can't remember something important.

I would say that it is generally unhelpful to contradict someone with dementia, to keep telling them they are wrong or bringing up a fresh loss. While the person may not remember the correct information they are being told, they can still experience the emotion associated with it. As we all know, a strong emotion doesn't subside straight away.

Can't go forward, can't go back

Professor Muireann Irish's research shows that memory isn't just for recalling the past; memory exists to help us learn and make sense of the world, and it allows us to plan for the future. Memory puts the world in context. Memory is also how we define ourselves: son, daughter, mother, father, job role, friend.

Memory helps us to anticipate pleasure. The memory of my morning cup of coffee certainly helps me look forward to the next one and gets me out of bed. We need memory to imagine, to plan. We use what we know about ourselves to make our lives better. Memory gives us imagination. With it we can imagine that if we just "do this," we will feel safer and happier, and experience more pleasure. Without that imagination, how do we find motivation?

Professor Irish has identified that some of the most distressing symptoms in dementia are anhedonia, the inability to feel pleasure, and apathy. Apathy, as we have noted previously, is often an early symptom of dementia and one that many carers find incredibly hard to manage. People lose interest in things that they used to enjoy because they can't anticipate the pleasure, so they don't have the motivation to overcome the inertia of sitting in a chair.

It is possible to help people with this apathy by taking the planning out or by bringing the enjoyment to them, like bringing grandchildren over for a visit. People with apathy might not show interest in starting an activity, but if someone helps them get started, they can become engaged and enjoy these things.

Apathy can be an extremely distressing symptom to caregivers, who might battle to push people to do hobbies, to do household tasks, or, at the extreme end of the spectrum, even to wash. It's hard to work out how much this bothers the person with apathy. There is some evidence from qualitative studies that it can cause distress, but in more advanced dementia it is hard to know if apathy is more of a problem for the person with dementia or for those around them.

Behavioral and psychological symptoms of dementia (BPSD)

When I feel stressed or edgy, I go for a walk. It clears my head and helps me burn off a stress response. If someone with dementia is in the hospital or a nursing home and goes for a walk—like our walker at the start of the chapter—it can be considered unsafe. Staff worry they will fall, the environment is filled with obstacles, and to the wanderer the rooms all look the same so they can end up in someone else's room. The normal human behavior of walking becomes a problematic behavior.

Our behaviors are constrained by what we consider cultural and social norms. If I suddenly found myself in a new group of people who lived in a very different place, I might find it very hard to understand the rules of what is and is not acceptable. We learn the rules of our own societies as we grow up.

One of the common reasons people are referred to see a geriatrician is because of "behavior" problems. Sometimes these behaviors are a manifestation of distress, sometimes they are a perfectly normal human thing to do but they are a problem in a particular environment. The label "behavioral and psychological symptoms of dementia" (BPSD) is an umbrella term for agitation, psychosis, and depression or disinhibition.

So often these behaviors come from a place of people trying to make sense of the world, but they can still cause very significant distress to caregivers. If someone wakes in the night and, in trying to make sense of their world, follows their usual pattern of what to do when they wake up (get dressed to leave the house), then this can lead their caregiver to severe and unsustainable sleep deprivation. A person with dementia might spend a day following their partner around because they love them and feel better when they are with them, but continually ask the same question again and again. These behaviors can be mild on the spectrum of challenging behaviors, but they nevertheless test the patience of their caregiver.

Troubling behaviors very often occur in the context of an unmet need or discomfort. Sometimes it is pain, as in the case of a man I saw who was described as "agitated." He had a blister from an ill-fitting shoe and did not have the words to describe the pain or the problem. At other times it can be a room that is too hot or too cold or a reaction to an unfamiliar caregiver who is perhaps in a rush. Even the issue of poor sleep can have an underlying unmet need. I've seen many people for this problem, but when I have examined them they have shown signs of cardiac failure. They can't sleep because they are short of breath when they lie down.

One simple strategy to minimize agitation in dementia is to try to avoid things that trigger a person. If one of my patients in the hospital is medically stable and hates having their blood pressure checked, we can just stop checking it. However, there are some things that can't be avoided, and one is personal care. It is generally okay for people to only shower once or twice a week, especially if the process causes a lot of distress, but continence management has to happen far more often. Many people with dementia are understandably very distressed by this. I would also be very distressed if a strange person tried to join me in the shower or take my pants off and I didn't understand why.

It is really important for caregivers to explain things to the person with dementia and to engage them to do as much of the task themselves as they can. Having a consistent caregiver help with these personal aspects of care can help, ideally someone of the same gender. Sometimes it is trying a new approach: a person who refuses disposable continence aids that look like diapers might wear absorbent underpants.

So, who actually has the problem?

I was asked to see Victor to manage his "inappropriate" behavior. Victor was in his late eighties, tall, still strong, but he had few words left. He couldn't tell me anything about his life. I learned from his family that he had been a general handyman who was always fixing and tinkering. He had been a warm and loving father and husband. Victor's family had tried hard, as many families do, to keep him at home, but they couldn't provide the twenty-four-hour care he needed.

At the facility he went into, Victor was labeled a problem. His behavior was called "inappropriate" because he wouldn't wear trousers. When I went to see Victor, it was immediately apparent why he wouldn't wear pants—he had a large hernia that extended into his scrotum, which made trousers very uncomfortable, so he took them off, having forgotten the learned social norm that we should be dressed. This "inappropriate" behavior had one of the easiest solutions I have ever come up with: get Victor a skirt. Victor was comfortable, and the staff were no longer uncomfortable.

What's important to consider with this is who exactly had a problem. There is nothing inherently wrong with being naked. Some societies are far more comfortable with it than others. Being uncomfortable with nudity is learned behavior. It is highly likely that in earlier years Victor would also have been mortified being naked in public, but right now Victor was just trying to solve the problem of physical discomfort. Victor's behavior was labeled "inappropriate," but it was really a problem for the other people around him. And it was a problem that could be fixed by thinking from Victor's perspective.

The most intense time of life

I walk into her room. She is in bed, wearing a hospital gown, the sheets pulled up. She cradles the baby with so much tenderness and love in her eyes. She looks up at me and smiles. I ask if it is a boy or a girl, and she tells me they don't know yet, they haven't unwrapped the baby. I am reminded of the moments I first held my own babies, the powerful rush of feeling, something beyond love at immediately meeting this baby and knowing he or she is the center of the world.

Except she isn't a new mother. She is an elderly woman with dementia. She has been very agitated recently, and then she was given so much antipsychotic medication that she couldn't move properly. She now has pressure sores on her fragile heels. I can see she is now reliving one of the most intense memories of her life. The memory of holding her new baby has been brought back with a doll.

When I call her daughter to speak about how her mother is doing, the daughter weeps. She says it's humiliating that her mother is reduced to playing with dolls. I feel her grief and distress at losing the mother she knew, but I also think to myself, what a beautiful gift to be transported back to one of the most intense, profound, and happy moments we can ever have in life.

Decreasing distress

When I see a patient with behaviors that their caregiver finds challenging I will always trial behavioral strategies and education, but there are also times when the person with dementia is suffering extreme distress or they are a risk to the safety of others because of aggression. Sometimes there are no obvious triggers, or the troubling behaviors really are symptoms of the disease itself, like paranoia.

There can also be risks to the safety of the caregiver in these cases. I have met many family caregivers, and even more people who work in assisted living facilities, who have been hit by someone with dementia. It's important to remember when this happens that the aggression is usually a manifestation of fear, such as when the person doesn't understand why a stranger insists on following them into a shower and strikes out. There are also some people for whom this behavior is the continuation shown over a lifetime of a trait toward aggression. Realistically, a slight woman in her late eighties poses very little threat; where aggression is particularly difficult to manage is in men with younger onset dementia. I have personally felt fearful of some strong male patients who are quick to aggression.

It is distressing for everyone when there are significant safety issues, not least because things like continence and personal care still need to be attended to. Some caregivers will need to learn to step away from their loved one if they are distressed. Some people with dementia will need sedating medication. It is only a small minority of people with dementia who are in this category, but there are still not enough specialized services to give them the help they need, and this can be a very difficult problem for caregivers to manage.

Delirium is not a UTI

The referral was to understand why Dorothy kept getting urinary tract infections (UTIs). When I got to the assisted living facility, I asked what sort of symptoms Dorothy was showing, whether it was pain on urination, burning, stinging, frequency, new incontinence, etc.

Dorothy was displaying none of those symptoms. What staff were noticing were recurrent episodes of delirium.

The day I visited, Dorothy was having one of her episodes. She couldn't hold a conversation, and she kept plucking at invisible things in the air. I looked through Dorothy's urine test results and saw there was not a single one with evidence of infection. Every time Dorothy became confused, someone would "diagnose" a UTI, then give her antibiotics. Unfortunately, they never actually checked if their diagnosis was correct.

Dorothy was greatly affected by these episodes and was becoming more frail with each one. After speaking to Dorothy's family and primary care physician, it seemed most likely to me that these episodes were actually seizures. I started Dorothy on an antiepileptic medication and the episodes of delirium stopped. Unfortunately, this was not until after she had experienced irreversible cognitive and functional decline.

While UTIs can cause delirium, it is not nearly as common as people think. Far too often I see people "diagnosed" with a UTI, and then everyone stops investigating. One of the key messages in geriatrics is to always take delirium seriously and to always keep a broad mind and consider multiple contributing factors before settling on a diagnosis.

How to make sense of it all

It is really hard to write about an experience that I will never be aware that I am having. While there are some people with dementia who are very active in the advocacy space—I have listened to their public talks and read things they've written—I have not interviewed them. They don't need me to speak for them, and as people who have maintained a high functional status for a long time, they are outliers.

While I was getting ready to write this chapter, I watched the excellent BBC documentary *Dementia & Us*, about people with dementia who were able to consent to be part of the program. They were followed for two years, from 2019 to 2021. It is an incredible journey by brave and generous people, who want others to understand their lives. The documentary showed families struggling, people's cognitive disability worsening, and caregivers realizing that they just couldn't look after their loved one anymore. We also see love, laughter, connection. We see the importance of the "living" part of living with dementia.

It also really brought home to me that what I see as a doctor, those all-too-brief consultations, is only a snapshot. It's often not even a snapshot of real life. It's a photo of people who have put on their best clothes, styled their hair, and are smiling for the camera, no matter what is going on at other times. Like a curated Instagram feed, I see the highlights selected for me.

While it is my job to try to see through what has been enhanced, I am very conscious that I am not seeing the full picture.

Ni de aquí, ni de allá—not from here, not from there

Suzanne Finnamore wrote: "Dementia is a place where my mother lives. It is not my mother." A person with dementia is exactly that: a person. Dementia does change people, but life changes people too. Some people with dementia will have a significant personality change, especially those with frontotemporal dementia, but for many, the lifelong continuum of personality, well, continues. For so many people, the good and bad experiences of life continue to shape them in dementia, and this is an important aspect of care. We can visit the person with dementia and meet them where they are in that moment. This takes a huge amount of compassion and empathy.

Aren't you all lovely?

The geriatric care unit during the COVID-19 outbreak was not a pleasant place to be. It was one of the oldest parts of the hospital, with five or six people to a room. All the staff were dressed in N95 masks, face shields, and gowns. We could hardly recognize one another, so I am sure we were indistinguishable to the patients, yet every time I spoke to Mary she kept saying how lovely we all were. Beyond a bit of lethargy, Mary was one of the lucky ones and sailed through COVID-19 in the pre-vaccine era. Her short-term memory loss meant that she couldn't remember what was going on, but she had the most incredible ability to see the good in any situation and to be happy.

I spend far too much time with people experiencing distress with dementia because they are the ones who need help, but when I think of Mary, I remember that some people with dementia are happy. They have the sunny ability to see the good in the world and are happy people. It makes me want to practice this skill in my everyday life.

Even someone with advanced dementia can still get enjoyment out of life. It is often through the simple, essential things, like touch and music. We all spend our days trying to have the best day possible and helping them to do the same is the greatest gift we can give someone living with dementia.

QUESTION 12:

How should I care for someone with dementia?

Sally

That promise, that stupid promise. Stella's mother had always said to her, "You're not putting me in one of those homes; promise me you'll never put me in one of those awful places. I want to die at home." Of course, when Sally made Stella promise, neither of them had any idea what they were agreeing to. Sally's own mother had died when she was fifty-five. It was a short illness, requiring only a few weeks of care. Sally had done it for her mother, and she had always expected Stella to do it for her.

Sometimes, when Stella got up for the fourth time in the night to assure Sally that the babies really were okay, she could go back to bed and recall with regret the one time she yelled at her mother that she was the baby, that she didn't even know her own daughter. Her mother had drawn back, terrified.

157

People told Stella she was a saint. They didn't see Stella's burning resentment at what her life had become. The last time she'd tried to take a shift at work, her mother had put a metal bowl in the microwave and nearly started a fire. So now she couldn't even afford to go out for coffee.

People didn't know about the dark thoughts, about what would happen if she just gave Mom too many sleeping pills and got a pillow to make sure it was really done.

Most people also didn't see that her mom was still her mom, that there was still love and joy to be had. They didn't see the times when Stella would play Dusty Springfield or The Seekers, and they would dance and sing; even though her mother couldn't often find words, "Georgie Girl" was still alive in her memory.

Stella loved her mother, but it was the relentlessness, the loss, the profound sleep deprivation that meant that sometimes the love did not feel like enough. She knew she was doing the right thing by her mother, but she also knew that she would never, ever make her children promise not to put her in a nursing home.

The superpower of humanity

Humans are capable of doing many bad things, but the thing that is less newsworthy, that is all around us, is just how incredibly caring we are. There is no other animal that can live in such large groups that has the abstract thinking for large scale cooperation. While history (and the present) is notable for wars and violence, the majority of human life takes place in the between times that don't make the news, when we live peacefully, caring for others.

Caring for others, performing acts of love, and in turn forming connection, is one of the most profoundly meaningful and rewarding things we can do in our lives, but even when caring for my own children I have moments of resentment when the demands are overwhelming. Sometimes all I want is to have time to myself, to clear my head, without a background barrage of demands.

We don't acknowledge nearly enough just how rewarding caring for other people is. We also don't acknowledge nearly enough just how hard it is. Caring can be incredibly good for our well-being, but it can also be very bad for our health.

We all care

With advanced dementia, particularly, some of the caregivers are likely to be paid professionals. These people, mostly women, do invaluable and essential work that is literally life or death but with incredibly little respect or pay. But much care is also provided by informal caregivers. This is the term we use to refer to unpaid workers such as relatives, friends, and neighbors who provide care to an older person with dementia. The care they give often goes beyond what is normal in the context of those relationships, such as a neighbor cleaning up a mess or a relative assisting with the bathroom.

Some informal caregivers receive additional support from formal caregivers, many do not. In the United States, there are around 11 million people providing unpaid care to someone with dementia.

This has implications for the future physical and financial health of these caregivers. Over a lifetime, women are likely to be paid less than men, and have often taken time out of their careers to look after small children, meaning less opportunity to save in a 401(k) and advance their careers. Unpaid caring work can further reduce opportunities for paid work. The group that pays a particularly high price for caring are "sandwich caregivers," those who care for two generations, particularly if they live with the person they are caring for. In the Australian Longitudinal Study on Women's Health, which is a twenty-five-year follow-up of 57,000 women who participate in regular surveys, around 25 percent are caring for two generations: one above and one below. Providing good care for people living with dementia means acknowledging that the well-being of their caregivers is a critical aspect of this.

Caregiving for someone with dementia can be incredibly stressful. People with dementia have preferences and rights, which should be supported, but it can be hard when the caregiver and the person living with dementia have differing perspectives on their care needs. I have met so many people who sit in my consultation room telling me that they do everything for themselves, while their caregiver sits behind them vigorously shaking their head. Some caregivers can become very isolated. I've heard from many people that those who they thought were their good friends have just about abandoned them when they learned about the dementia diagnosis. Some caregivers even become isolated from their own families.

I think one of the aspects of caring that we don't acknowledge nearly enough is that the small household of two older adults living by themselves is a very new phenomenon. Historically, most people did not get old, and young people far outnumbered the elderly and frail. When people tell me, "In my family/culture, we look after our elderly," they are missing the point that human society has never been structured like this. This century is the first time in human history that most people will reach very old age. For the rest of human history, there were far more children and young adults than older people, and few people were lucky enough to live into very old age. This demographic shift is wonderful but brings new challenges.

I have met a lot of people who feel like they've failed when they have to place their loved one in residential care, but I have never met anyone who didn't do everything they could, who didn't use every physical, emotional, and financial resource they had available to delay this. I see people who are burnt out, depressed, who can't remember when they last had four hours of unbroken sleep. One aspect of dementia care that I think people struggle to accept is that it is okay to get help, and it is okay to take a break. One strong recommendation I make for the caregivers of people living with dementia is to make a plan for respite care. Many people don't want to get this, because they plan never to use it, but you can't be entirely sure what the future will bring, and sometimes having your loved one go to residential respite for a week or two can make all the difference to avoiding burnout and allowing you to keep caring for longer.

A long loss

After seeing Helga in the nursing home, I led her daughter Elsa to a quiet room where I could tell her that I think her mother is close to death.

Elsa cried, repeating that "it's just so awful" again and again. Elsa wasn't grieving because the end was coming, she was *relieved* the end was coming. She was grieving because of what her mother had lost: her defining feature, her fearless intelligence. Now she was in a padded chair, immobile, unable to feed herself. She looked at her friends who could still call their mothers when something troubled them, whose mothers could still go out with them to the ballet and cafés, and celebrate family events. She felt an overwhelming sense of loss that this was gone from her life.

Nearly every caregiver I interviewed for this book cried when they spoke about how much they miss the relationship they used to have with the person with dementia. Unlike a clinical consultation, I did not have a time limit, and I was able to let people lead the conversation. A common theme was how much they loved the person with dementia but also their profound sense of loss. It has made me more conscious than ever how hard it can be for people to get the emotional support they need. I think that it is important for people to get support, but also to acknowledge and validate when someone is experiencing grief.

There are different types of grief. There is anticipatory grief at what *will* happen. Grief can also be ambiguous. When someone dies, there is often relief that their suffering is over but also a deep and profound sadness for the person who has been lost.

Grief and depression are not the same thing. Grief is a normal part of life—an awful part of life, but very normal. There is a spectrum from grief to depression. For some people grief will trigger a low mood that needs medical intervention. Around 20 percent of caregivers for people with dementia have depression. People who care for someone with depression also have higher rates of complex grief after the person they love dies. But there is also harm in pathologizing sadness. It is important to acknowledge grief and to validate these feelings.

Hello, beautiful!

Anne's husband, Geoff, doesn't walk anymore. He needs help with all activities of daily living, but whenever she arrives at the nursing home he greets her the same way he always has.

Thirty years after his dementia diagnosis, Anne is beyond grateful that he still knows her. When I met Anne, and she told me about her marriage, one of the most striking things was that she and Geoff had such an equal, loving, and supportive partnership. I would say that the majority of older people I meet have marriages with defined gender roles. Anne and Geoff have a truly modern marriage in which both supported each other in their careers.

Geoff's symptoms of dementia started when he was around fifty. He has frontotemporal dementia, so he showed significant behavioral changes. Anne found Geoff's changes incredibly difficult. At times, she feared for her safety, and with Geoff's disinhibition he would sometimes hit out when frustrated. He also developed road rage but insisted on driving.

With the support of her children, Anne did everything she could to keep Geoff at home, but it reached a point where Anne was too exhausted. She just couldn't enjoy life. She also couldn't work out what was wrong with her.

Anne had burnout.

Anne eventually made the decision to find an assisted living facility for Geoff. She knows she hasn't failed; she knows she did everything she could. Yet I meet a lot of people who think they have failed when their loved one goes into assisted living.

One of the things I've noticed about people with burnout is they don't know they have burnout. They can't see that they need a break and to temporarily let go of their responsibilities, that they need to share. I definitely see that lack of awareness when people have been shouldering a heavy burden for a long time. They can't see a way for others to help.

It is really important to remember that you need to meet your own needs. Caring is a marathon, not a sprint, and seeking out support can make all the difference, even if it is just speaking to other people who are going through a shared experience. There is no failure in using things like respite in assisted living to take a break—or even go on a vacation—to rejuvenate, get some sleep, and do something fun. Breaks such as this can make the difference for caregivers to be able to keep going.

Caring can also have a negative financial impact. It is very important to acknowledge that caregiving is gendered, so this disproportionately impacts women. For women in their fifties and sixties, caregiving can come at a critical time when they need to be saving for retirement. Restricting work opportunities can greatly increase the risk of financial insecurity. These are not easy problems to solve, at least not without addressing pervasive issues around financial inequality between men and women.

Having seen a lot of overburdened, depressed, and financially stressed caregivers, I would never tell my children not to put me in assisted living if I have dementia. I may enjoy it; I may not; but I don't want to put them in a position where their own health and well-being is compromised.

What is love?

It's important to have some self-awareness to accept help, to remember that humans evolved to live in complex interconnected societies where we help one another and it is deeply abnormal for one person to do it all by themselves.

It is also important to have a degree of acceptance as the caregiver, to acknowledge the need to meet people where they are. It is perfectly reasonable to find things stressful and hard.

There are interventions that can decrease caregiver stress and help people understand and have strategies to deal with distressing behavioral symptoms. If these were more widely available, life for caregivers of people with dementia would improve.

The aged care royal commission

The praise that caregiving gets is incredibly superficial in the context of how poor the pay is.

In 2018, an Australian TV show *Four Corners* aired a program about the problems in assisted living. In a breach of privacy for the woman and staff in the residential care facility, a resident's family had installed a secret camera. The camera showed her waking early and waiting for hours for staff to come and get her out of bed, which required two people and a hoist. It is distressing to watch this woman, helpless and alone. The staff, low-paid, hardworking women, who did not even have their voices disguised, were given the blame for the time it took to attend to her.

What the program didn't show is what goes on with staffing in assisted living overnight. There may have been only two staff responsible for a hundred people. They may have been dealing with multiple situations, with one person buzzing for the toilet while another had insomnia and was wandering into other people's rooms, yet another was sick, and another had fallen. The program didn't show that the workload of the staff was enormous, that finding time for two people to spare the twenty minutes each to get one person out of bed could be impossible. These hardworking women, earning around $23 an hour (about US$15), were not the problem. The problem was that their employers would not pay for enough staff to get through the work.

Many assisted living facilities are actually owned by large corporations that have the goal of making a profit. This is fundamentally incompatible with providing the best care possible for some of the most vulnerable people in our society.

During the aged care royal commission in Australia, which produced a report titled *Neglect*, there were two main groups whose voices were missing: people with moderate to severe dementia, and the casual caregiving workers, for whom taking the time out to provide a submission to the royal commission came with a risk to financial and job security that was just too high.

Many of the people who work in assisted living are migrants. The job is incredibly hard because the companies try to maximize their profit by having as few staff as possible. There is often barely time to give patients basic care, but they do their best. Many are also subject to racist remarks from residents and their families.

The National Aged Care Workforce Census and Survey in 2016 showed that there were almost a quarter of a million assisted living workers employed in Australia, and of those 180,000 were community caregiver workers or personal caregiving assistants, and around 47,000 were nurses. There are no mandatory staff-to-resident ratios in assisted living. A certificate III in assisted living takes roughly eight months, including 120 hours of placement. One hundred and twenty hours is not nearly enough time to understand the complexities of dementia care.

Staff are often casual workers who work across multiple facilities because they simply do not make enough money working at one facility alone, or they can't get a regular job. If you have a casual job, you can't easily speak up in the media, and you can't speak up at an aged care royal commission. You can't complain about racism or managers who berate you.

While the general public was shocked, I don't think any geriatrician was surprised when COVID-19 took off like wildfire in assisted living facilities, not after all the influenza and gastroenteritis outbreaks we had worked through.

During the outbreaks in assisted living facilities in 2020 and 2021, residents didn't just die of COVID, they died of neglect. In the outbreak at St. Basil's Home for the Aged, forty-five residents died of COVID, and five died of neglect after all regular staff were furloughed without adequate staff to replace them. Neglect means being left without food, water, or hygiene. It's unsettling.

I have read the report by the aged care royal commission, and I don't know if assisted living is fixable. At a very rough estimate, around 80 percent of people in assisted living have dementia, and while some can speak for themselves, many can't. Some people go into assisted living and actually thrive. The structure, routine, activities, and social meals can make a positive difference for them. Others struggle with this environment. If you need to wait for two staff members to be free at the same time to take you to the toilet, you might be waiting a long time.

Unless you work in a job like mine, it is easy to forget about older adults in assisted living. It's easy to shut them away, perhaps with some temporary outrage about COVID-19 infections, and then go back to forgetting.

The institutional model of assisted living has advantages: it has efficiencies of scale, and it fulfills a much-needed caregiving requirement. If institutions were shut down, there would be a huge caregiving deficit. While I support deinstitutionalization in theory, in practice I just don't think it's feasible. Assisted living needs to be funded properly, and those funds must be used transparently; it needs defined staff-to-resident ratios, and a recognition that caregiving is a skill, so people need training and appropriate pay. If assisted living continues to be run for profit, I don't see how this can ever happen.

We should all care

I don't know anyone who doesn't have a caregiving relationship in their life. There is a deep and profound satisfaction from doing things for others, especially when the other gives back with thanks or even just smiles.

I wish caregiving was more visible and valued. I wish that it wasn't so undervalued just because it is mostly women's work. I wish it wasn't so badly paid. I wish that we had a more communal society where it was everyone's role to care.

Caregiving work is a skill: it is learned. Caregiving for people living with dementia, whether paid or unpaid, does not get nearly the recognition and respect it deserves.

QUESTION 13:

Do people with dementia have the capacity to make decisions?

Dolores and Bruce

Dolores gave him that smile, the one that was only for him. Bruce sat on the bed next to her and leaned in for a kiss, just a peck, but she opened her mouth and her tongue found his. Her hands were on his shirt; he shivered at her touch and pulled her close. Her hands moved down to his pants, and he felt himself harden. He reached up under her dress; she opened her legs and moved closer to him. He moaned her name—and then suddenly the door was wide open, a nurse standing there with an accusing glare, the one that says, "You know you're not supposed to do this."

Bruce and Dolores met at church, so he was surprised that first night when she invited him in, reached up to his tie, pulled him close, and kissed him. When they met, their children were all adults, so there were no worries about condoms or missed pills. It was just fun. Their children thought their relationship was silly and called them lovesick teenagers. Her daughters tried to talk her out of marrying him.

Five years after they met when Dolores's memory started to go, they still had *this*. She still reached for him, gave him that knowing smile, pulled him close. The day her daughters made him put her in the nursing home, when they said he couldn't look after her, he went home and cried. When the doctor said she didn't have the capacity to consent to sex, he did not agree. She couldn't say his name, but it was the look she gave him, the smile that had always been there, the way she reached for him.

From the day they were discovered by the nurse, Bruce was never allowed to be alone with Dolores again. They even had a doctor examine her genitals for signs of damage. A nurse sat either side of her, holding her hands down because Dolores wanted to stop the strange man looking at her.

After that day, when he could only sit with her in the large common room of the nursing home, the TV blaring, people chatting and dozing around them, always with watchful eyes on him, Bruce felt humiliated knowing that people thought he was a sex pest and not a loving husband responding to a wife who still knew him in that most intimate way.

Consenting to sex

Consent to sex has become a hot topic in the media, and there is an understandable focus on teens and young people, but being able to consent to sex is also an issue in dementia patients. Consent should be freely given, and to give it, someone needs to understand what and who they are giving consent to. The idea of enthusiastic consent is consent with body and words, positive affirmations, not just "giving in." Just because someone consented to the last sexual encounter does not mean they consent to the next one. Consenting to one sexual activity, like mutual masturbation, does not mean a person consents to all sexual activity. Consent can also be withdrawn at any time. Some states of Australia have introduced affirmative consent laws, which make it the responsibility of people in the act of having sex to make sure their partner wants to do it too.

To be able to consent, you also need to have the mental capacity to do so. This means knowing and understanding what you are doing and who you are doing it with, knowing the implications, and knowing that you can stop.

A person with dementia who thinks a man is her husband, even though he is not, is not able to consent. In nursing homes, this can present an additional layer of complexity. If two people with dementia each think that the other is their spouse, and they enjoy cuddling and get comfort from this, meeting an essential human need, is this really a problem?

The complexity of capacity and consent also stretches beyond sex.

Decisions, decisions

I met Carl after he had broken some bones falling off a ladder. When I asked him about his medical history, he told me to just look at his hospital record because he had also been admitted a few months earlier after falling off another ladder. My personal judgment was that Carl should have stayed off the ladder after the first fall, but this was not Carl's view. He had judged it was more important to clean the gutters before the expected rain. I advised him not to do this again, but it is also up to Carl as to whether he follows the advice. Carl is an adult who does not have dementia. He has a right to make these decisions, even if I personally think that climbing a ladder you recently fell off is a bad idea.

We all make all sorts of decisions all day long, like what we spend money on, what we eat, what job or activity we fill our days with. We occasionally make very big decisions, like buying a house or investing money with that family friend who seems really trustworthy. Just because someone makes a decision that we consider risky or dangerous does not mean they lack capacity.

A small child has very little autonomy over their life. Their parents choose their house, clothes, food, school, and, to a large degree, who they socialize with. Once someone is eighteen, they are legally an adult and can make decisions about getting married, voting, and drinking alcohol (in Australia), even though people's brains aren't completely mature until they are in their twenties. It is also not true that children are incapable of all considered decisions; there is a gradual increase with age.

One of the fundamental underpinnings of society is the idea that people have a right to make their own decisions. We don't take away people's rights just because they make decisions that someone else would consider bad. If you look around, you can see that almost every individual will come to a different idea of what a good decision is for them. The other side of this is that I don't know anyone who bases all their life decisions on being safe and healthy at all times.

While every adult can make their own decisions, if we're being honest, a lot of people don't always make what I consider the "best" decisions. Even I don't always make the best decisions. (Do I really need another pair of shoes? No, but I'll buy them anyway.)

The right to make decisions comes from the ethical principle of autonomy.

Capacity

Capacity is a concept I spend a lot of time with. It means being able to understand and make a decision. For someone to have capacity, they need to be able to do the following:

- Understand the information relevant to the decision and the effect of the decision.
- Retain that information to the extent necessary to make that decision.
- Use or weigh that information as part of the process of making the decision.
- Communicate the decision and the person's views and needs as to the decision in some way, including by speech, gestures, or other means.

Capacity is also specific to the decision that needs to be made. As an example, a person with dementia may have the capacity to decide to have sex with someone, but they may lack the capacity to decide to marry them. Someone with dementia may have the capacity to appoint an enduring power of attorney but not have the capacity to manage their own money.

Every country will have different rules, but in most places, there is an assumption that all adults have capacity unless proven otherwise. We assess capacity only if there is a trigger, such as someone with dementia wanting to make a major decision, like where they live. If I have a patient and we recommend assisted living and the patient agrees, there is no need to assess capacity. If they don't agree, and we can see no other option, then we commence the assessment. Placing someone in assisted living against their will is an option of absolute last resort because people have a right to make decisions in line with their own values, even if they lack capacity. When we reach this point, there is a legal process to follow that involves an application to a magistrate, who will require proof that there really is no other option. An example would be when someone wants to remain at home but lives alone and can no longer get on and off a toilet. They might not see that as a problem, but it clearly is for their general safety. Even if a situation is not perfectly safe for an individual, such as where there is a risk of falling, we will still try to support the person's wishes to remain in their circumstances.

Branka

The worst thing about being in the mental hospital was the pills. Every morning, they had to line up at the counter to get the tablets, the ones that left Branka feeling like she was experiencing the world through a layer of honey. The nurses would watch her swallow them, one by one, then inspect her mouth. It was humiliating. Her doctor had sent her there because she couldn't sleep; now her sleep didn't feel like sleep at all, it felt like a heavy suffocating blanket that she could never quite take off, all because of the pills. She hated being there—the routines, the rigidity, the way she was supposed to talk about being sad to the very doctors who labeled her as insane because she was so sad.

When she finally got out, she vowed she would never go back again. She pulled herself together; she did the things a housewife and mother was supposed to do. Sometimes she even acted it so well that she felt okay.

No matter how many years after Branka had been in that asylum, she could never take pills without a rising wave of nausea. When she got diabetes and high blood pressure, she refused to take any pills. The doctors came again, they tried to pry into her mind, they tried to trick her with questions about what she remembered, questions about her home. All Branka knew is that she would never go back to that loony bin again.

By this time, Branka needed support to stay home because of her dementia. Branka's case manager, Katherine, was worried about her staying home because she would only intermittently let caregivers into the house and never took her medications. Katherine suggested that Branka should go into assisted living to make sure she took her pills. Legally, however, this is not the least restrictive option and does not fall in line with Branka's previous wishes. If someone does not take their pills when they have capacity, that is their choice (again, even if this is not what their doctor recommends). If they develop dementia, they may no longer have the capacity to make this decision, but if it is in line with previous values, in this case Branka being extremely distressed by pills, then this needs to be part of the decision-making.

Living dangerously

One of the most difficult things with dementia is that, as it progresses, people can need help with everyday activities but lack insight into the help they need or other risks. Falls are a common example. People with dementia are more likely to fall, and if they have osteoporosis or fragile bones, this can result in disastrous fractures. Some people with dementia may have a falls alarm but forget to use it. This can leave families extremely worried about their loved one who lives alone. We live in a risk-averse society. Risks of falls, risks of not eating, risks of fire. We also have an increasing proportion of people who live on their own, rather than in a multigenerational household, where help is available from the people you live with.

For many people, their home is also exactly where they want to be. A home is so much more than a residence: it has comfort, memory, freedom. Assisted living is set up for scale. All meals come from a limited menu at prescribed times, activities are within the range set by the facility, your shower is the fifteen-minute slot from the time the caregiver arrives at your door, bedtime is determined by when the day shift changes to the night shift with the lower staff ratios.

Some people thrive on the routine and structure of assisted living, but for many this is exactly what they don't want.

Even when people have dementia, for most of the illness they still have wants and priorities. It is absolutely undeniable that someone with dementia who wants to live in their own home but needs help with showering, eating, and cleaning—often while denying they need this help—is relying heavily on a caregiver. I often have to sit with the exhausted son or daughter of a patient and tell them that we haven't tried the least restrictive option, so their loved one has to go home with additional services, like personal care, even if the person with dementia will only intermittently let them through the door. I have huge sympathy for the strain this puts on the caregiver, since the reality is that supporting the person with dementia to live the life they want can also put huge constraints on their loved ones.

Dementia and driving

The consultation started badly. Roger was very mad at the last geriatrician he saw and wanted to tell me all about it. He was furious that this doctor had told him he needed a driving test to continue driving. I listened calmly, then I confirmed that he did indeed need to have a driving test. I have also been the doctor who has made someone so furious they never want to see me again because I told them about their legal obligation to tell the road authorities about their diagnosis of dementia. In such a case, it's the end of our therapeutic relationship.

Of course, I always try to deliver this news calmly and with empathy, but driving is such an emotive topic, so associated with independence, and so essential if you live in a suburb with poor walkability or other transport options, that it can be a huge blow. Some people will even tell me that their life is over when they can't drive.

There are people with dementia that can drive safely. Other people can drive safely in familiar areas and may have a conditional license. While there are cognitive tests we can do in the clinic to work out whether someone is likely to be able to drive safely, which include assessing vision, reaction time, and motor skills, and I can ask questions about car accidents, near misses, or mysterious scratches and dints on the car, the only way to really know is an on-road driving assessment with an occupational therapist in a special dual-controlled car.

A diagnosis of dementia does not automatically mean losing your license; it usually means needing annual tests to assess driving, because dementia is a progressive condition. As a doctor, I can't take someone's license away; only the roads authorities can do that. I can notify the roads authorities if I think there is an immediate risk to safety, such as their family telling me that they are extremely unsafe.

One of the most important principles of practice is that I recognize that people have a right to make the decisions that are in keeping with their values and priorities, even if they aren't the safest decisions, like someone who lives alone who is at risk of falls. But driving is where personal freedom can meet problems with public safety. We've all been on road trips with that sense of freedom, adventure, and escape. What we don't stop to think about is that a car is also a deadly weapon.

Stop reading and do this now

This information is general advice only, as legislation differs between states and countries.

Have you appointed a power of attorney and made a will? If not, the first thing I want you to do when you stop reading is contact your friendly local lawyer and get these done. An enduring power of attorney is someone who is able to make financial and lifestyle decisions on your behalf if you lose the capacity. They can also make decisions about where you live and getting help in the home. Importantly, they are legally obliged to act in line with your wishes.

A medical power of attorney allows someone to make medical decisions, such as consenting for surgery if you are unconscious or if you lose the capacity. If no one has been legally appointed, there is a hierarchy of who is responsible for making decisions. If the treatment is urgent for lifesaving purposes or to relieve extreme distress (such as when a paramedic treats someone who has been in a car accident), no consent is required.

The actual legal wording will vary between jurisdictions, and it is important that you find information relevant to where you live. Having this in place before you actually need it is key, because it can be quite the legal process to sort out once you have lost your capacity, often involving an expensive formal assessment and application to a legal tribunal to have someone appointed as the power of attorney. Since this is something I never want to put my family through, I have already appointed a power of attorney, which would be enacted should I lose capacity.

The next important thing to do is to have a conversation with the appointed power of attorney about your wishes and values, especially for the person tasked with medical decisions on your behalf. Importantly, the financial power of attorney can only use your money for your needs, not to take themselves on a fancy vacation.

When someone loses capacity and doesn't have a power of attorney, it can create a significant legal and logistical problem for the family. Things like accessing money to pay an electricity bill or needing to sell a house to pay a bond for assisted living become impossible.

When I am assessing someone's capacity to appoint a power of attorney, I will ask whether they understand what a power of attorney is, whether they know what powers it gives, and who a suitable person would be. The suitable person needs to be someone willing, available, and able.

You may choose to appoint one or many people as your power of attorney, and they can act jointly (all must sign for everything) or severally (each can act independently). For older adults with older spouses, it is often a good idea that at least one power of attorney is someone younger, like an adult child.

Making a will is another essential part of being an adult. To be able to make a will, a person needs to have testamentary capacity. In simple terms, they need to understand the assets they have and who should expect to receive them after they die.

These legal things are time-consuming and a little unsettling but absolutely essential to do before you need them.

A note on elder abuse

When my grandfather had dementia, he used to pay for everything with $50 notes and tell people to keep the change. At this time, he was losing the ability to understand numbers and money. He could still remember that $50 was a lot of money, and this would cover most things, but he wanted to hide the fact that he didn't really know the detail of how much something cost and what change to expect.

People weren't consciously taking advantage of my grandfather, they just thought he was a generous old man, but since he didn't know the value of money he was at risk of financial abuse.

Financial abuse is depressingly common for older adults with and without dementia. It is also just one form of abuse. Abuse can be physical, emotional, sexual, or through neglect. In Australia, we don't know how big the problem is, but overseas estimates range from 2 to 14 percent of older adults, rising to almost 40 percent in assisted living, are abused in some way. The majority of elder abuse happens within the family, and women are more at risk than men, and sons are more likely to be perpetrators than daughters. It is heartbreaking to see this in action and to imagine that this abusive man was once his mother's precious little baby boy. People are vulnerable to abuse from those they trust and depend on for care.

Estimates of the prevalence of elder abuse come from people reporting the abuse to authorities. This means they are likely to be far lower than the reality, especially for people with dementia. Some people with early dementia would be capable of reporting abuse but not if their disease is advanced. Often people who are dependent on others for care cannot safely report the abuse. I've had many instances where multiple siblings in a family are accusing the others of abuse, and we have no way of knowing who is doing what.

The most common abuse I see is neglect. I remember one woman with multiple pressure areas, whose neglect must have been chronic and awful. She would have been suffering for long periods, unable to get help. She must also have been isolated, and her caregivers were possibly isolated also. I don't know whether she had dementia or not—she was too close to death when she came to the hospital. Abuse thrives when the victim and the caregivers have little to no social support and no formal support. Often elder abuse occurs in the context of complex family dynamics, and sometimes someone who is the perpetrator was once the victim. Sometimes there is a dynamic of control, where the parent controlled the child well into adulthood, shunning outsiders, and now the child as an adult continues to shun outsiders, even though the care is beyond them.

Abuse is often far more banal: the caregiver who breaks with frustration and yells at the person they love. This emotional abuse may well not happen if the caregiver has the support they themselves need.

Elder abuse is yet another way that family violence thrives within shame and secrecy, and open conversation and community support are key to preventing it.

Bringing it back to capacity and consent

One of the myths about appointing an enduring power of attorney who can make financial and lifestyle decisions is that it will take away independence. Often, it is the opposite that is true. One example is the person who wants to stay in their own home but isn't able to organize people to come in and help. If they have appointed an enduring power of attorney, once they have lost capacity that person can organize caregivers and access home care packages to support their independence.

An awful lot of people I meet say they haven't made a power of attorney or will because they don't need it yet. An enduring power of attorney only becomes active once someone loses capacity. It is really unpleasant to think about lacking the cognitive capacity to make decisions. I think this is why so many put off these important legal tasks and difficult but important conversations. What is important to remember is that when you are making an enduring power of attorney, you are ensuring that the right person is going to be making decisions on your behalf if you lose the ability to do so.

Should people with dementia be able to choose end-of-life options for their future selves?

My first job as an intern was working on a surgical ward. My co-intern and I would do an early morning round with our registrar, then he would go to the theater, and we were left to do all the ward jobs for the patients, like inserting intravenous drips.

Clive was just shy of ninety and had been admitted for a bowel obstruction, which had been relieved by an emergency operation to remove a cancer. After the surgery, Clive was extremely confused and would pull at the various tubes connected to his body, which were giving him fluids and antibiotics. Every time his drip came out, usually with a splash of blood, someone would have to hold Clive down while one of us interns replaced it. Clive didn't know why he was in the hospital, he didn't know why people were hurting him with needles, so he tried to fight us off. I was trying my best to help him survive, but restraining someone and causing them pain still felt wrong.

These memories of forcibly inserting needles flashed into my head when I read about the case of a seventy-four-year-old woman with dementia in the Netherlands who was held down by members of her family so a doctor could give her a lethal injection. The lethal injection was to fulfill the wishes of an earlier iteration of herself.

Years earlier, after her diagnosis with Alzheimer's disease, she had written this:

> I would like to use the legal right to be given voluntary euthanasia, when I think the time is right. I do not want to be placed in a nursing home for elderly people with dementia. I want to say goodbye to my loved ones in a timely and dignified manner. My mother in her time had been in a nursing home for twelve years before she died, so I have close experience of it. I know what I am talking about. I definitely do not want to experience this, it has traumatized me severely and really saddened the whole family. Trusting, that when the quality of my life is so low, that at my request euthanasia will be performed.

The problem was that by the time she moved into assisted living, which she had nominated as her predetermined time when she wanted to have euthanasia, she no longer understood this decision, and it was not clear whether she wanted to live or die. Her doctor at the assisted living facility assessed her and saw that she was in great distress, with the loss of dignity that she had so feared. Wanting to act in accordance with the woman's advanced care directive, and after extensive discussion with the woman's family, her doctor made the decision to proceed with euthanasia without asking the patient what she wanted.

The case made international headlines because the doctor faced criminal charges, although he was ultimately acquitted.

While my initial reaction was to remember how distressing holding patients down to inject them was for me as a doctor and for the patient, I also understand that the doctor and the patient's family were trying to act according to her wishes. She had a clear idea in advance of what life with late dementia would be like and did not want that for her future self. Her doctor and her family were endeavoring to support her autonomy.

Advanced dementia and death

Dementia is a progressive, terminal neurological disease. The life expectancy after diagnosis is usually around eight to ten years, although this varies significantly.

I am not going to lie: the idea of living with advanced dementia is scary. In our society, most people with advanced dementia are cared for in assisted living. This is because their care needs are usually beyond what can reasonably be provided at home. In the advanced stages of dementia, familiar muscle patterns are lost so people have trouble with walking and swallowing. People lose functional language and cannot always communicate wants, needs, and discomforts. Some people become completely nonverbal. People also have trouble eating. They can have difficulty chewing food and swallowing and can aspirate food into their lungs. And when people die with dementia, it is usually because they have pneumonia.

There are signs that someone with dementia is approaching end of life. One of these is getting recurrent pneumonia. Pressure injuries are also predictive of the end approaching, although with careful nursing these are preventable. Some people will start to lose weight for no obvious reason. Once I've established that there are no easily reversible problems, these symptoms are the trigger to have a conversation with loved ones about impending death.

"I'm sorry, but your mom is approaching end of life."

At work, I talk about death a lot. When I see a patient with advanced dementia, even if it is a routine review, I start a discussion about end of life with the family.

This conversation can go a few ways. Sometimes, people are shocked. Some people do not know that dementia is a terminal disease. Some haven't been able to mentally engage with the inevitability of death at all.

This is, however, unusual. More commonly when I tell family that their loved one has reached a terminal stage of dementia, they are almost relieved that someone is saying what they had been thinking. This means taking important steps to prioritize quality and comfort. One thing that makes this easier on the person responsible for making decisions is if there has been a conversation earlier, often years earlier, about what the person with dementia would want.

In these situations, I also have the responsibility as a doctor not to offer futile treatments. I won't offer CPR, or intubation in intensive care, when

I know from research and clinical experience that in advanced dementia, these are not going to prolong life.

How do you make an advanced care plan?

For someone early on the dementia journey, or even someone without dementia, this chapter may have suggested the idea that it's time to make an advanced care plan. An advanced care plan is a document in which you record the values you want to guide decisions in the situation that you are unable to make your own decisions regarding your medical care. One of the problems with advanced care planning is envisaging and recording the many potential medical problems and treatments. A better way to go about creating your plan might be to record what is important to you. Would you want medical treatment if it meant you ended up unable to talk or walk? Is it more important to preserve your life, even if there is only a small likelihood a treatment will work and a high risk that you could end up in a nursing home? These are difficult questions to answer, and the answers might change over a life span. Right now, I have young children, and I would take any chance to stay alive for them, but I know that many of my patients who have reached very old age don't feel that way, and I know that once I reach very old age, I might feel the risks and discomfort of a certain treatment outweigh the potential benefits.

Good palliative care

One of the phrases in medicine that makes me cringe more than any other is when a doctor says, "There's nothing we can do." What that doctor means is that there is nothing within their skill set to fix or cure the disease. However, even when this is the case there is always something that we can do.

One of the most important things we have in life is the ability to make decisions to bring pleasure and enjoyment to ourselves and others. We choose foods we like, we spend time with people we enjoy seeing, we do fulfilling activities. This is the essence of palliative care: having the best day we can *today*. This will mean different things for different people and will alter over the stages of an illness.

The goal of palliative care is to prioritize enjoyment and quality of life above all else, and this includes avoiding futile medical treatments.

What does a good death look like?

Looking after people at end of life and seeing their families gather has been one of the greatest privileges of my career. It is incredible to see the love someone has generated in their life. For adult children and grandchildren with busy lives, it is a rare opportunity to just sit and be together. Even in the saddest of times, I see people taking joy in being with people they love so much.

Of course, the other part of a good death is controlling symptoms. Symptoms at end of life can include pain, agitation, and shortness of breath. When someone is dying, they lose interest in food and fluid. Good palliative care involves managing these symptoms.

Some people worry that when their loved one is on morphine it is hastening their death. While a large dose of morphine will kill anyone by stopping their breathing, it is worth keeping in mind that there are people who spend decades dependent on opiates. When we prescribe morphine in terminal care, we aren't trying to stop someone breathing; we use small doses to manage pain and shortness of breath. While morphine is helpful for anxiety, we also commonly prescribe benzodiazepines (medications like Valium) to help with agitation. We also use antinausea medications and sometimes medications to dry oral secretions.

Even at end of life, we think people can still hear, so playing music and speaking are likely to give comfort. Just simply holding someone's hand can give profound comfort. When people can't eat or drink, we give mouth care, and often families will assist and have a swab and some water to keep their loved one's mouth clean and moist.

It can take a few days for someone to die, even when they are no longer conscious. During this time, they will need management of continence and regular turning to prevent painful pressure sores.

When people are dying, they usually become increasingly drowsy until they cannot be roused. Breathing can become irregular. At the end, many will have Cheyne-Stokes breathing, which is an irregular breathing pattern with rapid breaths, followed by a pause. People can develop gurgly breathing due to secretions in the throat. This sounds distressing, but it doesn't cause distress to the person dying and can be managed with medications.

While most people want to die in their own home, the reality is that good end-of-life care is hard work and takes considerable skill. Some families are able to do this at home, often if members can work in shifts and with palliative care support, but nursing homes, hospitals, and palliative care wards have the staff, equipment, and skills available for this type of care.

For people in residential care, many prefer to die in their residential care facility rather than travel through a hospital emergency department in the last days to hours of life. By the time someone with dementia enters residential care, they may or may not be making their own medical decisions. When someone goes into assisted living, it is important to make an advanced care plan in line with their wishes. Many people (or their substitute decision-maker) feel that it is in the person's best interests to avoid emergency departments and have treatment in their facility whenever possible. In Australia, many hospitals are able to support this, with programs that have nurses who can visit assisted living facilities to provide additional support at end of life.

Artificial feeding and dementia

"If I'm ever stuck eating mush, I want you to shoot me."

Food and entertaining had been the center of Mario's life. He had worked for years as a food writer and was a respected restaurant critic. He had always said to his son Matteo that if he couldn't eat real food, he didn't want to live.

As his dementia progressed, he and Matteo kept up their weekly restaurant dinners, but eventually he found it easier to just visit the same restaurant that was owned by old friends. They were always so kind, even when Mario called multiple times to confirm the same booking. Mario was a proud figure as he walked through the restaurant, in his well-cut suit, still discerning about his food but not remembering it was the same dish he'd eaten last week.

Many years after his diagnosis, Mario fell and could no longer walk. Reluctantly, Matteo found a nursing home for him. At the nursing home, the speech pathologist told Matteo that Mario had a weak swallow and he needed soft foods. Matteo remembered Mario's words, but when he lifted the spoon, Mario would see it and open his mouth.

Matteo felt conflicted. This was exactly what his father had said not to do, but he had opened his mouth. Was this going against one of the most important things Mario had ever asked of him?

Food is for fun

I don't think that there is nearly enough emphasis given to the importance of food to quality of life. Most people cannot imagine enjoying a life without their favorite foods.

My colleagues who are older than me remember using tubes to feed people with advanced dementia. A nasogastric tube is a tube that is inserted in the nose and goes down the throat into the stomach to provide nutrition (I hesitate to call the pale-brown liquid "food"). Another method of feeding is a percutaneous endoscopic gastrostomy (PEG), for which a person is sedated and a doctor performs a gastroscopy, placing a camera into the stomach, then inserting a tube through the skin until it can be seen inside the stomach and secured for feeding.

In line with the American Geriatrics Society, I do not recommend these for my patients with advanced dementia. This is because they do not meaningfully prolong life or improve quality of life. And even if someone is having supported feeding, they can still aspirate their saliva and get pneumonia, and there is also significant risk of death from the surgery to place the PEG tube.

In all advanced diseases, when a person is approaching end of life, they lose their appetite and interest in food. This doesn't mean they are dying of malnutrition: they are dying of the disease itself. When someone is at this stage of dementia, it is important to refocus on food as a form of enjoyment and emotional connection rather than reducing it to calories. If the person with dementia is quite drowsy but enjoys a few spoons of coffee, ice cream, or custard when they are awake, then focus on that enjoyment, not whether these foods are meeting their nutritional needs.

In the jurisdiction where I live, medical practitioners are not obliged to offer futile treatment. Substitute decision-makers are also not allowed to refuse palliative care. Since hunger and thirst are distressing symptoms, if a person is alert enough to open their mouth when they see a spoon coming, I would interpret spoon-feeding as palliative care.

This is the problem with making plans for a future self. The future self may no longer go along with the plan.

The then-self now-self problem

"I thought it through once again last night, from start to finish and back, and in the end this is what I want. Purely for myself. This is what's best for me."

Annie was in her home, surrounded by her family. The night before they had been to a favorite restaurant. Annie felt that her dementia was already impacting her quality of life, and she wanted to die before it got any worse. Her doctor gave her a lethal sedative to drink. A few hours later, he gave her a lethal injection. In the Netherlands, this is completely legal. Annie's current self was making a decision for her future self, but how do we know if her future self would actually have been happy?

There is also no escaping that some people with moderate to advanced dementia do not have good quality of life. Some experience fear because they don't know who they are or who their caregivers are. Some people will resist personal care, even when they are incontinent. Others experience distressing hallucinations and paranoia. Some people are in pain.

There are people who seem to have an innate joy that shines through, even when their memory is gone. They are happy to have people to care for them, they enjoy their food, and they are delighted with activities at their assisted living facility.

Some philosophers argue that personal identity requires psychological continuity. This would mean that a person with advanced dementia is no longer the same person, and this makes the preexisting wishes of their non-demented self null and void.

I don't agree with this.

Even in later stages of dementia, people are still the product of a lifetime of experience, habits, and happenstance. Even when nonverbal, people will still have preferred foods or might respond to a particular song. Even when they can no longer explicitly recognize their daughter or son, on an emotional level they respond.

Even within one person's journey with dementia, some treatments may be appropriate early in the disease but not appropriate late in the disease. I have had patients with early dementia, still living at home, for whom I have advocated to have a pacemaker for a slow heart rate that is causing them to collapse. For someone who is bedridden with advanced dementia, this isn't appropriate. An advanced care plan needs to change with the progress of the disease.

Before the sun sets

I don't know what it's like to experience advanced dementia, and if you are reading these words, neither do you.

I do know that there comes a point in the disease when comfort outweighs all. Once someone is bedridden and nonverbal, I do not recommend prescribing antibiotics if they aspirate and get pneumonia, because even if I successfully treated this episode of a life-threatening disease, I am only prolonging life for days to weeks. I cannot fix the devastating, progressive damage to the brain. I can prescribe medication to relieve pain, anxiety, and shortness of breath, and my nursing colleagues provide skilled comfort care.

I don't know if people should be allowed to decide in advance to undergo euthanasia at a later point in the disease. I certainly wouldn't want to hold someone down for a lethal injection. I also don't think I would enjoy living the final stages of dementia. Would I want someone to kill me when I was past the point of knowing?

I am in an unusual position in our society because I have seen this stage of dementia up close many, many times. I can make a more informed choice than most. When we ask people to make a plan for their future selves, or even ask the next of kin to make a decision, most only have scant knowledge to inform this decision.

In many jurisdictions where euthanasia is legal, people with dementia can't access it because they don't have the capacity by the time they only have six months to live.

If the legislation is expanded so that anyone with a terminal diagnosis can access euthanasia, will this have people rushing to death earlier than they would like for fear of the future? Will they miss spending quality time with loved ones? If legislation allows someone to choose a time in the future when they no longer have the ability to live independently in their home, this will differ hugely between people, depending on the symptoms they get or the level of support their family can provide.

In our society, death is hidden away. It becomes a "defeat," almost as though it is optional. If we are going to give people with dementia the gift of the best death possible, we need to start talking about it and acknowledging that death is one of life's few certainties.

Can improving diet help to avoid dementia?

If you are looking for quick diet hacks for dementia prevention, I am going to disappoint you. I might also make you happy, because I take a "most of the time" approach to healthy eating, not an "all the time." There is no one correct diet for dementia prevention. There is no one nutrient or superfood that will buffer the brain against aging. The right diet for brain health lies in a quote from the author Michael Pollan: "Eat food, not too much, mostly plants." When Michael Pollan said "food," he meant wholefoods like fresh produce, not the kind of food that takes up most space on the supermarket shelves.

Keeping your brain healthy is all about vegetables and variety.

You are what you eat

Our bodies are constructed out of the foods we choose to eat. Whether you eat a meal of frozen chicken nuggets made of ingredients you could never find in a domestic kitchen, or a piece of grilled fish with steamed vegetables, tiny molecules will be integrated into your cells and used as fuel for your body. Chemically, chicken nuggets and fish and vegetables are very different, and this is why the food you eat is important for your brain function.

Malnutrition is an ongoing, significant problem in our society. The kind of malnutrition I see most commonly isn't in people who look like they are starving; it is in people who are overweight or obese and have a diet that is lacking in the nutrients their body needs. At an extreme end, I have seen patients who are getting enough calories but who have scurvy from eating little in the way of fruit and vegetables.

It is a constant effort to try to choose the right foods for health, especially when our supermarket shelves are filled with cheap, palatable, packaged food-like substances covered in dubious health claims. To make this even more confusing, every other person seems to have an opinion on the "right" rigid and restrictive diet we should be eating, whether it's vegan, keto, paleo, or—and this is the one I find most outrageous—carnivore. It's enough to make you want to put it all in the "too hard basket" and eat a chocolate bar.

While reading nutrition research can make my head spin, especially with all the different diets, there are simple consistencies. Eating for your brain is much more about patterns of eating than single superfoods or rigid diets. It's about finding a way to make choices that are sustainable and enjoyable. It's understanding that it's about what we do most of the time, not all the time. We must also acknowledge that food is more than just calories; it has cultural and social meaning, as well as being one of life's essential pleasures.

Taking this approach provides a framework for eating that can benefit your brain health and keep the enjoyment in food (and life).

Body weight is a relatively simple measure of health, and by no means perfect, especially in a world where being thin is so socially desirable. People can have a body mass index above the "normal" range and still be very healthy. Indeed, for people ages sixty-five and older, it seems to be associated with longevity. At the same time, for people with a body mass index above 30, there can be health consequences.

Obesity is an incredibly complicated area, especially because being at a higher weight can be a source of stigma and discrimination.

The English Longitudinal Study of Ageing (ELSA) recruited 6,685 people who were ages over fifty and free of dementia at the start of the study, then followed them for up to fifteen years. During this time, researchers took measures like body weight and blood pressure, and did cognitive testing. They also measured abdominal circumferences. People were then divided into groups based on body mass index and abdominal circumference. Over the course of the study, 453 people developed dementia. People who were obese were around 35 percent more likely to develop dementia, compared to those with a BMI of less than 25.

There are multiple reasons that obesity is linked with dementia. People with obesity are more likely to have diabetes and high blood pressure. There is also the risk of conditions like obstructive sleep apnea. Fat tissue, especially around the abdomen, is metabolically active tissue that is associated with higher levels of inflammation. It may be that those higher levels of inflammation are causing changes in the brain.

Obesity is a risk factor for dementia but one that is incredibly difficult to tease out from other health aspects, since obesity is linked to sedentary behavior and a lower quality diet. Body weight is easy to measure—all you need is a scale. Lifestyle behaviors are not easy to measure. Unless someone is living in a laboratory, studies rely on self-reporting, and humans are very bad at remembering everything they eat and do. While the ELSA researchers did ask people about their activity levels (low activity was a risk for dementia), they didn't ask about dietary patterns.

The ELSA study isn't the only one to find an association between obesity and dementia. The link has been shown in many other studies. The question is what to do about it.

The rise of ultra-processed foods

When my grandmother was growing up, she ate meat and three vegetables for dinner (one of the vegetables was always potato). The milkman did daily deliveries. Instead of a fridge, her family had an ice chest, with ice that was also delivered. Food was different back then, and very few people were obese. Obesity rates only really started to rise from the 1980s onward, around the time that ultra-processed foods (UPF) started to hit the shelves.

Have you ever sat down with a box of crackers and found you finished them before you knew it? Have you then noticed that you are still hungry? This is because you are eating ultra-processed foods, which some people call food-like substances, that are designed to bypass the brain's sensors that tell you that you have had enough to eat.

Ultra-processed foods make up most of the middle shelves of the supermarket. They include instant noodles, supermarket bread, cake, crackers, and many breakfast cereals.

Diet culture has sequentially demonized various macronutrients. For years, fat was bad, especially saturated fat, so simply avoiding that could guarantee health. We have been told to avoid sugar and salt, to eat more protein. These simplistic instructions ignore the reality of being a human and the range of foods and combinations of nutrients we need. They have also fed into the ultra-processed food industry, with the creation of "low-fat" foods. A diet high in UPF contains little fiber, high amounts of sugar and salt, and multiple other ingredients that can be disruptive to the gut, like emulsifiers. Over the years, a lot of dietary advice has focused on avoiding one macro- or micronutrient, like saturated fat, refined carbohydrates, or salt. This doesn't reflect that our foods are made up of a combination of these. Personally, I think that this approach is confusing.

Food is a chemically complex substance. A banana is not simply one micro- or macronutrient. It is not just fiber or protein or vitamins; it is also yellow, a little sweet, soft to chew, and has a distinctive taste and smell.

If anyone is wanting to make a positive change to improve their health, the simplest approach is to stop thinking of food as calories and components and instead eat foods that are not processed, such as fruit and vegetables, or foods that are minimally processed, such as cheese and natural yogurt (not the low-fat sweetened yogurts).

Your brain on UPF

Ultra-processed foods are only a relatively recent food development, and there haven't been long-term studies linking it with dementia, although in a study of over 100,000 people, those who ate more ultra-processed foods were associated with a higher risk of cardiovascular and cerebrovascular disease.

Many of the studies looking at diet have been done in mice and rats. They have shown that rats who are fed a diet that is high in saturated fats have poorer memory function. There is also some human evidence. In a study of 105 university students who usually followed a healthy diet, the half that was randomized to change to a diet high in saturated fat and sugar had worse memory performance in just a week.

A diet high in fats and sugar is linked with depression, which can itself lead to a slowing of cognition and difficulty with memory. For some people with depression, changing diet to exclude UPF and instead include lots of vegetables, legumes, olive oil, and fish can improve their mood, a claim supported by a randomized trial of sixty-five people that ran for twelve weeks. The Royal Australian and New Zealand College of Psychiatrists also recommend instituting a healthy diet for people with mood disorders, while acknowledging this is only one aspect of management.

There is also evidence of long-term benefit from good nutrition. In a cohort in the UK of 459 people with eleven years of follow-up, those who ate more vegetables, fruit, and legumes, and less trans-fats, fruit juice, soda, salt, and sugar, compared to people on less healthy diets, had bigger hippocampal volumes. Hopefully, the healthier your diet, the healthier your memory is likely to be.

What are the diets that are good for your brain?

Multiple "diets" have been studied for their benefit to brain health. While research titles use the word "diet," what they are studying is really more dietary patterns. The diet that has been most studied is the Mediterranean diet. In a trial with 7,447 participants, ages between fifty-five and eighty, in Spain, called PREDIMED (Primary Prevention of Cardiovascular Disease with a Mediterranean Diet), people were assigned either a low-fat diet or a diet with lots of vegetables, legumes, fish, nuts, and olive oil. They actually stopped the trial early at 4.8 years because they found that the people on the Mediterranean diet had significantly lower cardiovascular mortality. A later analysis showed that people who followed this dietary pattern also had preserved cognition.

The other diet that has been extensively studied is the MIND diet. MIND stands for the Mediterranean–DASH Intervention for Neurodegenerative Delay (DASH stands for Dietary Approaches to Stop Hypertension). This has a lot in common with the Mediterranean diet but it also has a few important differences, in particular the focus on green leafy vegetables. There are fifteen components to the MIND diet.

Ten brain healthy foods
- green leafy vegetables
- other vegetables
- nuts
- berries
- legumes

- whole grains
- fish, poultry
- olive oil

Five less healthy foods
- red meat
- butter/margarine
- cheese
- pastries and sweets
- fried/fast food

What is so good about the MIND diet?

Following the MIND diet means eating lots of variety and flavor. A day's eating like this might mean porridge with berries for breakfast, a salad with leafy greens for lunch, and dinner of some kind of fish and vegetables, with some nuts to snack on along the way. Eating food on the MIND diet will have the following important components:

- **Fiber.** Fiber really is the unsung, humble hero of health. Fiber is the plant cell walls, the tough outer coating on plant cells that we can't digest, but our microbes can. Not only does fiber helps us to feel full, it helps our microbes to feel full as well. Our microbes break down the fiber to make molecules that are good for general health and brain health. Giving our gut microbes the fiber they need also protects the integrity of the gut barrier. Eating a variety of different vegetables and whole grains will give you the variety of fiber you need.

- **Polyphenols.** Polyphenols are chemicals plants make to protect their DNA, and in turn are good for us. There are more than 500 different polyphenols and various ones occur in every plant food, including herbs and spices. The way to get lots of polyphenols is to eat a big variety of food.
- **Healthy fats.** Food sources for this are fish, chia seeds, avocado, nuts, and olive oil.
- **Lots of micronutrients.** Different foods have different vitamins and minerals. Eating a variety of foods will provide all the different micronutrients you need for your brain.

A note on alcohol

I have met far too many patients who have dementia that is related to alcohol to think of alcohol as something good for the brain. While many studies have reported that moderate alcohol intake may be good for hearts and brains, there are often important confounding factors that accompany alcohol intake, such as socioeconomic status or other health behaviors. A study published in *The Lancet* in 2018 reported that, worldwide, alcohol was the seventh leading risk factor for death and disability-adjusted life years lost. Even if alcohol may provide some protection against cardiovascular disease, the increased risk of cancer more than counteracts this. People also engage in risky behaviors when they are intoxicated, and I have met too many people who have fallen after alcohol and sustained bleeding on the brain. Even the idea of moderate alcohol intake is a problem because so many people underestimate how much they drink.

When I take an alcohol history, I don't ask how many glasses of alcohol someone has; I ask how long it takes to get through a bottle of their preferred beverage because a standard drink is very different from the amount of alcohol most people pour into their glass.

The safest level of alcohol consumption for brain health is none, but many people do enjoy wine, including myself. I usually restrict myself to drinking one day a week, and only one to one and a half glasses. If you do choose to drink, I think it is important to have limitations on quantity and frequency.

If you have concerns about alcohol intake, I suggest contacting your doctor.

What are the micronutrients that are important for brain health?

Micronutrients are molecules that we need in our diet in small amounts. While the actual amounts are tiny (hence the name "micro"), without them our bodies cannot function. Deficiencies in these are also potentially reversible causes of cognitive impairment. As always, it is best to get these into your diet. If you have any concerns, see a dietician.

B12

B12 deficiency can cause anemia, unsteadiness when walking, and numbness in the hands and feet. People who are deficient in B12 can also develop dementia, and sometimes cognitive changes are the first symptom of deficiency. B12 is mostly found in meat and dairy, so people on a vegan diet are at risk of developing a deficiency in B12. Some medications, including common reflux medications, can interfere with absorption of B12, and there are people who develop an autoimmune disease whereby they can't absorb it. B12 deficiency can be diagnosed on a blood test and fixed with regular injections by a doctor.

Thiamine

Thiamine is also known as vitamin B1. It plays a key role in metabolic pathways. People who are alcohol dependent are at particular risk for thiamine deficiency because they often have poorer quality diets, and alcohol impairs absorption of thiamine. People who are deficient in thiamine can develop Wernicke-Korsakoff syndrome, which causes them to have trouble walking, abnormal eye movements, and extremely poor short-term memory. These symptoms also occur when someone is starving or experiencing anorexia nervosa. In the hospital, we prevent this by giving intravenous thiamine if we are concerned about alcohol intake or malnutrition.

Vitamin C

While we think of scurvy as something sailors died from in the age of exploration, in the large central city hospital where I work, I usually see a case of scurvy once or twice a year. It is often in people who are alcohol dependent and on a very poor diet, although one of my colleagues did once diagnose it in a young man who was living off convenience-store pies to save money. Vitamin C deficiency causes a red-purple rash, bleeding gums, pain and swelling in joints, and the hairs on the legs to be shaped like little corkscrews. Vitamin C deficiency can also result in cognitive slowing and depression.

Folate

Folate deficiency can also cause a decline in cognitive function. Deficiency in folate is rare because many foods are fortified with it. Blood tests are often not reliable, because folate levels go up quickly after someone eats a meal with folate.

You can't supplement your way to brain health

The shelves of my local pharmacy are absolutely full of supplements with dubious, nonevidence-based promises on their labels. They are selling the fantasy that if you just take a pill, your health will be improved. While it would be lovely if life was as simple as eating what you like, then taking a pill, the evidence is clear that it is far better to get your nutrition from food. Consider a supplement like fish oil, which is one of the most common supplements. Not only can the capsules be rancid, but in a randomized controlled trial in the USA, which compared these supplements to a placebo, fish oil capsules showed no impact at all on heart disease or cancer.

Numerous studies have reported that a higher level of fish consumption is associated with better brain health. There is an awful lot of difference between a capsule containing one specific chemical component of a food and a delicious piece of barbecued fish. It is likely that the whole fish package is good for the brain, not just one component.

In one case, a dietary supplement was promoted for brain health and memory function. In an analysis of three randomized controlled trials, there was no convincing evidence that the aid decreased the risk of progression to dementia or improved cognition for people with dementia. Since it was not a drug but a supplement, the makers were allowed to have on the label that it provides "memory support" and it could be sold over the counter.

When you are looking at the shelves of supplements at the supermarket or pharmacy, it is worth remembering that there is no legal requirement in Australia for the makers to actually have evidence that what they are selling does what it claims on the label. I understand the appeal of taking a supplement, it feels like an easy fix, but it in no way replaces the complex nutrition of real food.

Can exercise help to avoid dementia?

Here's the thing about exercise—it isn't just about dementia. Don't get me wrong, exercise is incredibly good for your brain, and there is very strong evidence that it can prevent dementia, but it is also a great example of just how interlinked brain and body health are. Basically, if you are fitter and stronger, so is your brain.

Compared to the vast majority of people who have lived throughout history, we really are in highly unusual times. For most of our human history we would have spent our days moving, just to keep about the business of staying alive. Rather than walking over to the fridge to get food, or ordering dinner on a delivery app, we would have had to walk, dig, climb, track, chase, and forage, or there would be nothing to eat. Exercise didn't exist because being sedentary simply wasn't an option if you wanted to stay alive.

Modern sedentary lives are so bad for us that according to the World Health Organization, 3.2 million deaths a year are caused by inactivity, and insufficient physical activity is the fourth-leading risk factor for mortality.

As an adult who is very active, I know that I feel at my best when I exercise. Exercise is an ingrained habit for me; I really don't feel right if I don't do it. But not everyone has the opportunity to be active. Exercise can be so hard to fit in as part of a day. Many people drive to work, or now work from home, and there can be so many commitments in life that it is hard to squeeze out the time to go for a walk. If you're not in the habit of being active, it can also be hard to overcome the feeling of inertia to start something new.

There is overwhelming evidence that exercise is good for your brain. It can protect your cognition as you age, but it is also excellent in the here and now to manage stress and improve learning.

How do your brain and your muscles talk to each other?

Our bodies are a constant state of cross-talk and communication. Whatever is going on in one part of the body, our brain needs to know about it, urgently. The majority of exercise involves large, whole-body movements, so of course our bodies need to know where to direct blood, whether extra oxygen is required, and how to get rid of the metabolic products of exercise.

When we exercise, we activate the sympathetic nervous system (the fight-or-flight response described in Question 9). This causes some blood vessels, such those to the gut, to constrict. It causes others to dilate, including those that carry blood to the skin, so we can end up red and sweaty. Our heart rates speed up, and a higher volume of blood is pumped out each time it contracts. Our breathing becomes faster, we take bigger volumes of air in and out, and our muscles demand more energy. Exercise also has a positive impact on immune-system function. While exercise initially stimulates immune activity (an evolutionary throwback, in case we are at risk of getting wounded), it also quickly turns it back off again, resulting in lower levels of inflammation.

Why is exercise so good for the brain?

Whenever I got stuck writing this book, I did some form of exercise, even if it was just a short walk. That is because I know that when I exercise, a whole raft of changes happen in the brain that make it work better. This is also likely why it is so good for dementia prevention.

When you exercise, there isn't just more blood going to the muscles, there is more blood going to the brain. There is also an increase in all sorts of "good" brain chemicals. One of them is brain-derived neurotrophic hormone, which stimulates the hippocampus and promotes brain plasticity. There is also a downregulation of inflammation and, in evidence from studies of animals, even positive changes in the gut microbiome.

Exercise also has positive short-term effects on cognition, improving memory and learning. Many guidelines, including those of the Royal Australian and New Zealand College of Psychiatrists, include exercise as a treatment for mild to moderate depression.

As we age, physical activity can help to maintain cognitive flexibility, memory, and attention. By keeping our brains as healthy as possible with exercise, we improve our chances of staying cognitively well into very old age.

What do the population studies show us?

There is overwhelming evidence from cohort studies, the kind that take a group of people and measure certain outcomes every few years, that the most physically active have a reduced risk of dementia.

One compelling study of exercise and dementia was a study that followed a group of women for forty-four years. The women were recruited in midlife, and their fitness was assessed by getting them to run on a treadmill. They were then tracked for many years. The fittest women had an almost 90 percent reduction in their risk of dementia, and even if they did get dementia, it was at a far later age than the less fit. The reason I find this compelling is that the researchers actually directly measured fitness and the long follow-up time is impressive.

Another study from Korea, which used data available from a national health insurer relating to people with a median age of seventy-three, asked people to self-report physical activity and then looked for a dementia diagnosis around three to four years later. This study also identified that people who were more active were less likely to get dementia, but a particularly interesting finding was that the decreased dementia risk started with even low levels of physical activity.

It isn't just cardiovascular fitness that is good for our brains: having more muscle in older age is also associated with better brain function. Multiple studies have found that older people with better muscle strength have better brain function. The reasons for this are fascinating and complex. Muscles and the brain talk to each other in many ways, and having a higher muscle mass can improve metabolism and protect against diabetes. As an aside, maintaining muscle strength is also key to healthy aging in general. Muscle strength declines with age, and this is a common cause of age-related disability and loss of independence.

It's probably not news that exercise is really, really good for you. I think that many people know this; it's just that there are a lot of barriers to putting it in place. So how much exercise do we need to do, and how do we actually get it done?

How do we get more exercise into our day?

The recommendation from the World Health Organization is that we should aim to do 150–300 minutes of moderate physical activity every week or 75 to 150 minutes of vigorous physical activity.

One hundred and fifty minutes a week is only twenty-one minutes a day of brisk walking. It doesn't sound like much, but data from the Australian Institute of Health and Welfare shows that only 45 percent of adults manage this, and that number reduces with age. Women are less likely than men to be physically active, with only 41 percent getting enough activity. In data from the Australian Institute of Health and Welfare, for those ages sixty-five and over, 69 percent of men and 75 percent of women were insufficiently active. When you look at the recommendation that adults should undertake strength training twice a week, it gets even worse, with only 23 percent of adults managing this. Overall, only 17 percent of men and 14 percent of women meet the guidelines for both activity levels and strength training.

The reality is that there are a lot of barriers to exercise in everyday life, including access to appropriate spaces. Many women, including me, don't like to exercise alone outside after dark. Life can also be extremely busy, especially at the stage when you might have small children and paid work. Some people are lucky enough to get incidental exercise at work, but a lot of people spend their days sitting at a desk.

There is also very little in the way of formal support. For many people who are sedentary in their forties and beyond, starting an exercise routine, beyond walking, needs some input from an expert, like a trainer. There is a very real risk of injury if you go from the couch to trying to play a game of basketball or lifting heavy weights at the gym. Technique and a gradual start are both important. Additionally, if you don't have the right financial resources, this can be a challenge.

So how to get started?

As noted, the recommended amount of exercise is 150 minutes a week at moderate to high intensity, with two sessions of strength training. Moderate- to high-intensity exercise means working hard enough that it becomes difficult to carry on a conversation.

When people ask me what the best form of exercise is, I say that it is the one you enjoy and the one that is accessible. This seems like a simple statement, but there is a lot to unpack. Gym classes can be expensive, and some people have specific needs, such as when they are recovering from injury, while other people will need the motivation of friends.

Finding the right exercises, ones that are fun and enjoyable, really does make life so much better and has the side benefit of being great for long-term health.

What are key strategies to get started with exercise?

- Find something you like to do.
- Put it in your calendar.
- Work out with a friend.
- If you can afford it, find an exercise physiologist or experienced trainer who will help you slowly and safely build up your strength.
- Try committing to a class at your local gym.
- Focus on how good you feel afterward.
- Try an online program at home if you need to build up some confidence.

An ideal week of exercise is to do 150 minutes of moderate- to high-intensity exercise, and to include two sessions a week of strength training. Here is the most important thing to remember: don't let perfection get in the way of getting some exercise done. Walking is free, can be social, and almost everyone can do it. If you try to walk at a speed at which it is hard to have a conversation, you're getting a workout. If you can add in some strength training through weights or yoga, fantastic.

QUESTION 17:

Why are challenge and rest so good for our brains?

We have all heard the phrase "use it or lose it" in relation to our muscles, but it is just as true for our brains. If you decide to spend the rest of your life sitting on the couch passively watching TV, your brain will only need very limited connections.

Luckily, life is full of ways to challenge your brain, which are often enjoyable and surprisingly easy to find. A simple dinner with a few friends is enough to keep your brain mobile.

Why is socializing so good for our brains?

For the vast majority of us, being isolated and disconnected feels bad, which makes sense from an evolutionary perspective. A human on their own just could not survive life as a hunter-gatherer, or even as a subsistence farmer. In the industrialized world we live in, it is possible to get food, drink, and shelter with little help, but this is just existing, not really living. There is a reason why being put in isolation is considered an extreme punishment, even in the jail system.

Social isolation is also very bad for our cognition. Solitude is a lost opportunity for cognitive challenge, as staying home all day with your own thoughts means one less way to exercise your brain. We learned much about social isolation during the time of COVID-19 lockdowns. Not only was it distressing, it also meant fewer chances to flex our social muscles. Anecdotally, I have seen many people with dementia who deteriorated when they lost their regular opportunities to socialize.

How can we get more social?

My five-year-old happily tells me he is friends with every person in his class. Every day he goes off to school and gets to do collaborative activities in the classroom and on the playground. Children expect to make new friends, and they aren't shy about getting to know others. Classrooms are also an easy place to do this, with teachers making an effort to focus on the social development of their students.

As an adult, it's not so easy. Dinners get planned and postponed and "we should get coffee" promises aren't followed up. The things that held us together, such as school, university, or work, can fray when life gets busy with careers and children. This can get even harder in older age when people retire. If that loose group of office acquaintances isn't replaced, social circles can become sparse.

The "how" of improving your social connection is going to differ for everybody, but a good place to start is with something you enjoy. If you are reading this and don't feel connected enough, just remember there are other people who are in the same position. It is daunting to do something such as join a new club or start a new hobby, but other people will be there for exactly the same reason.

What about brain training?

Isn't it an appealing idea that you can sit on your couch and tap away at your tablet or phone, all the while protecting yourself from dementia? Brain training apps appeared a few years ago, with cute little logos like a brain lifting weights. If exercising your brain this way sounds too good to be true, it's because it probably is. While there is evidence that using brain training apps will make you better at brain training apps, this has not yet been translated into gains in everyday life. One study, called the ACTIVE Cognitive Training Trial, randomly assigned 2,832 people with a mean age of 73.6, showed that people who received small-group in-person training in reasoning, rather than memory or visual processing, had slightly less decline in their ability to do important daily tasks, but the effect was tiny. Around a third of the participants were lost to follow-up, which can mean that the sicker people, who may have been more likely to have cognitive deficits, dropped out.

There is unlikely to be harm from doing brain training, but it's a false sense of security to think that an hour on a game means you can spend the rest of the day sitting on the couch eating potato chips and keep your brain healthy.

An enriched environment

In studies of laboratory mice, those living in an enriched environment had higher levels of neuroplasticity. I'm not entirely sure how to translate an enriched environment for a mouse to a free-range human, but one way to enrich your environment is through work.

A surgical colleague in his sixties asked me once about whether he should start brain training. I pointed out to him that his job, diagnosing and treating patients and working in a team, was already providing him with excellent cognitive engagement. A stimulating, enjoyable job is good for challenging your brain. Basically, if you are working and enjoying your job, you're already doing "brain training."

For people who don't find work challenging, or who have transitioned out of paid work, the list of leisure activities that have been studied and found to have an association with a decreased dementia risk is extensive. One study measured thirteen different activities, including knitting, exercise, visiting friends or relatives, and going to restaurants. Doing more leisure activities was associated with a lower risk of developing dementia.

These studies are hard to interpret, and it is really important not to confuse causation with correlation. It is entirely possible that losing the ability to do lots of leisure activities was an early sign of dementia. The way I interpret this sort of study and apply it to my life is to think about the importance of doing things I enjoy. Many leisure activities are things we do to add more fun to life. Joining a language class may protect you against dementia, but it is also fun to do for its own sake.

Protect your senses

Our brain's primary role is to interpret and integrate sensory information to assist us in navigating the world to stay alive and reproduce. Sensory information, including sights and sounds, gives our brain information and stimulation. There is good evidence that hearing loss is a risk factor for dementia. This makes sense because with hearing loss, there is less stimulation coming in and therefore less engagement with the world. It is also a good reason to get your hearing checked and get hearing aids if you need them.

Sleep

Some world leaders have famously boasted of how little sleep they need. Personally, I would feel much more confident in a leader's decision-making if they were adequately rested.

Not only does lack of sleep feel awful, but it is also linked with almost all of the diseases we are most likely to die from, including dementia.

What does your brain do while you are sleeping?

Although we aren't moving around, or seemingly doing anything active, our brains are almost as metabolically active when we are asleep as when we are awake. There are two main phases of sleep: slow-wave sleep and rapid eye movement (REM) sleep, which is when we dream. Our brains cycle through these two phases throughout the night. Earlier in the night, we spend more time in slow-wave sleep, and later in the night more time in REM sleep.

During slow-wave sleep, slow electrical impulses spread like, well, a wave through the brain, as though the neurons are being resynchronized. During this phase of sleep there are also changes in blood flow, which means the glymphatic system (the system that circulates the fluid around the brain) is able to clear out the metabolic waste of the day.

During REM sleep, the brain's electrical activity looks very different. This is the phase when we dream. We are also mostly paralyzed during REM sleep, which is lucky when you consider how crazy our dreams can be! We only spend around 20 percent of the night in REM sleep. During this phase, the brain's electrical activity looks like a sawtooth pattern. There is a theory that during REM sleep, our brains are able to integrate information from different parts of the brain, improving creativity and problem-solving.

How does missing sleep cause dementia?

It is worth taking a moment here to talk about one of the difficulties in researching sleep and dementia. When I am speaking to someone who may have dementia and a person who knows them well, I always ask about sleep because changes in sleep, including insomnia and vivid dreams, can be symptoms of dementia due to damage to the parts of the brain that control sleep–wake cycles.

Researchers and doctors are often left wondering if the sleep problem is a symptom of dementia or a cause. One important study can help shine light on this question because it includes decades of follow-up. The Whitehall cohort study, conducted in the UK, has 7,959 participants and has been running for thirty years. The researchers have analyzed sleep at age fifty, then looked at dementia diagnoses years later via an electronic health record. People who reported less than seven hours sleep a night were around a third more likely to get dementia. The researchers also did an interesting sub-study in which they gave some participants wearable sleep recorders. At the time of publication this group had only an average of 6.4 years of follow-up, but the data showed that those who slept less than seven hours per night had a higher risk of dementia.

It makes a lot of sense that if our brains don't have time for all the critical reset functions they need to perform, like waste removal and repair, then we get immune dysregulation and a buildup of damaging molecules.

How do we improve our sleep?

As I'm sure many of you are aware, being sleep-deprived is immediately bad for your brain in so many ways. When we haven't had enough sleep, we are less able to make new memories and regulate our emotions; we become more impulsive and worse at problem-solving. Just ask anyone who has ever indulged in a spot of online shopping after a night shift.

Every animal sleeps. While you only have to wait one night to start experiencing adverse effects of sleep, over the longer term being sleep-deprived is very, very bad for you.

As anyone who has done shift work will know, there is no easy way to shift between day and night. People who regularly do shift work miss around ten hours of sleep per week, due to day-to-night transitions, with serious health implications. In a study of nurses, those doing more than three night shifts per month had a small increase in the risk of cardiovascular death. Shift work has also been listed as a possible carcinogen by the World Health Organization.

Ten hours sounds like a lot of sleep to miss, but if you stay up an hour later watching TV for one week you've already missed seven hours.

Ten steps to improve sleep

1. Get up at the same time each day.
2. Get out for some daylight early in the morning.
3. Take regular exercise to make sure you are physically tired and to burn off any excess stress hormones.
4. Avoid caffeine after midday. This means no tea, coffee, or energy drinks as they take around twelve hours to leave your system.
5. Eat an early dinner, then no snacks. Going to bed overfull can worsen reflux.
6. Choose a regular bedtime. Ideally, around eight hours before you plan to wake.
7. Don't spend too much time in bed. Bed should be for sleeping and sex, so we don't have psychological associations with wakeful activities (other than with your intimate partner).
8. Have a wind-down routine. This can mean reading a book with a cup of herbal tea or meditation in a dark room. Best to not argue with strangers on the Internet.
9. Keep the light low before bedtime. Too much light will stop your brain producing sleep chemicals.

10. Choose sleep. It is very, very easy to find reasons to stay awake, and most of them are not worth it. Even if you are in the middle of a really good TV show, it will still be there tomorrow before your chosen bedtime.

When I am speaking with people about making positive lifestyle changes, my recommendations usually come as a bundle. However, if someone is not getting enough sleep, this is the place to start. While sleeping pills are very popular, they quickly stop working and over the long term they actually worsen sleep quality. The most evidence-based way to improve sleep is through lifestyle strategies. We all have a natural circadian rhythm. Working with this is the best way to get the eight to nine hours the vast majority of us need to function at our best.

The key takeaway from these discussions of sleep, exercise, nutrition, and cognitive challenge is that what is good for our bodies is good for our brains. While our brains really are remarkable organs, they are still made of cells that are interacting, directly or indirectly, with everything else going on in our bodies. If you want to improve your long-term health, you don't need to choose an organ to focus on or a disease to avoid. For the most common chronic diseases—whether dementia, heart disease, or diabetes—the same lifestyle steps will reduce the risk of them all.

QUESTION 18:

How can your doctor help you prevent dementia?

There is a lot of prevention that you can do on your own, but not all. In medicine, many specialties are for one particular body system. If you have a blocked artery in the heart, the cardiologist will unblock it; if you have one in your leg, the vascular surgeon will unblock it; and if it is in your brain, the neuroradiologist will do the job. They are all arteries, they can all have the same buildup of fatty inflammatory plaque, but a different specialist will treat each different location.

It's probably confusing and is the result of one of the most unfortunate truths of medicine: it's all about fixing what is broken rather than preventing the problems in the first place. This also impacts the research space, where most disease outcomes are studied separately, even though they are all caused by the same underlying cellular and biological processes, whether it is diabetes, heart disease, or dementia.

Basically, every organ needs a good blood supply, and if this is compromised, the organ, whether it's heart, brain, or kidney, will start to fail. This leads us to heart health.

Under pressure

The blood supply to all these organs is highly regulated. Systolic blood pressure refers to the pressure created when the heart muscle contracts to circulate blood around the body. Diastolic blood pressure is the pressure when your heart is relaxed. When your doctor checks your blood pressure, systolic is the top number and diastolic is the lower number (for example, 120/80) measured in millimeters of mercury (mm Hg). Both numbers are important. Systolic pressure is the amount of pressure to get blood to all the organs, including the brain. If someone has hardened arteries, this pressure will need to increase. Diastolic pressure is the pressure when the heart relaxes, and this is when the heart actually gets its own blood supply. If the blood pressure is too high, it can lead to damage to the blood vessels. If the blood pressure is too low, organs, especially the brain, don't get enough blood.

Since this is so important, we have a combination of neuronal and hormonal mechanisms to regulate blood pressure. The carotid baroreceptors in the neck can detect if the pressure drops and a message is sent to the heart to beat fast and with more blood with every contraction, and for the blood vessels to constrict. If our blood pressure drops, our kidneys experience less blood flow and activate the renin-angiotensin-aldosterone system of hormones that acts to increase blood pressure by conserving salt in the blood and constricting peripheral blood vessels.

When blood supply to an area increases, it can make that part of the body swollen (the most obvious example is an erect penis). Since the brain is housed in the skull, which is a fixed container, an increase in volume due to increased blood is very risky. Conversely, while other parts of the body can get by temporarily with a reduced blood flow, like the tips of our fingers turning white in the cold, the brain cannot. If someone has a critical lowering of blood pressure, like after the loss of a large volume of blood, blood vessels to other parts of the body, including the gut, will constrict to preserve blood flow to the brain. This means that blood supply to the brain is tightly controlled to account for the daily fluctuations that can happen in life.

There are some primary causes of high blood pressure, such as a hormone-producing tumor, but these are quite rare. The most common type of high blood pressure is called "essential hypertension." The thing about having high blood pressure is that unless it is extremely high (systolic, somewhere above 200), there are no symptoms. You can go about your life with a blood pressure well above 130/90, and the first symptom is a catastrophic stroke, whereby part of the brain loses its blood supply, either due to a blood vessel blockage or a bleed. It is so important to get your blood pressure checked because treatment to keep it in the optimal range is excellent for brain health. The caveat for this is in the patient group I see most: the oldest, usually defined as ages eighty-five and above. By the time people reach this age, there is far less evidence for the benefits of tight blood pressure control, and this needs to be balanced with other risks from medication, such as falls.

While we have an excellent understanding of the long-term impact of high blood pressure on cardiovascular risk and dementia risk, we still don't completely understand why this happens. One clue is that in small studies of people who are living a hunter-gatherer lifestyle there is no increase in blood pressure with age, so it might be something about the foods most of us eat or not being active enough.

It is important to know if you have high blood pressure by getting it checked by your doctor, because then you can start on medication to get it to a healthier level, and this can make a big positive difference to long-term brain and heart health.

Like branches of a tree

The largest blood vessel in the body is the aorta, which comes off the heart. Blood vessels spread out and branch all over the body, right down to the smallest blood vessels called "capillaries." These blood vessels are just wide enough for one red blood cell to squeeze through, and this is where the exchange of oxygen and carbon dioxide takes place. It's not entirely clear what initiates hypertension, but once it has started there is blood vessel remodeling that then drives more hypertension. This means that these blood vessels can't easily dilate if there is a need to increase supply. There is also a loss of the smallest blood vessels, so the tissues they supply get less oxygen. While having high blood pressure for a short period of time won't do damage, in the long-term it means there is less blood supply for the body, which is particularly critical for our energy-hungry brains.

As we learned earlier in the book, certain functions are related to certain anatomical areas of the brain. If a blood vessel to the part of the brain that controls movement is blocked, it will lead to a sudden and dramatic medical event. If the blood vessel goes to a part with a less obvious function, like the part of the brain that controls personality, it is possible that no one immediately notices. You would be surprised to learn how many people have had strokes and are not aware of them. Over time, high blood pressure also damages the capillaries—the blood vessels that are critical for suppling oxygen and nutrients. This damage will not be apparent straight away, but eventually it builds up and affects how well different parts of the brain talk to one another, which can lead to trouble recalling memories and processing complex information.

Keeping your blood pressure in check, along with lifestyle management strategies like exercise and a good diet, is essential for keeping your brain healthy. It is also important to check with your doctor about one of the conditions that commonly goes with high blood pressure: diabetes.

Diabetes

Our cells need a constant supply of glucose, but like many things, too much is not good for us. Our bodies have careful regulatory systems to ensure that the glucose levels in the blood remain at just the right level. If your blood glucose gets too high, cells in the pancreas called "beta islet cells" detect this and release insulin. Insulin is a hormone that works like a key to a door, and lets glucose into the cells, thereby reducing levels in the blood. Without it, the glucose can't enter the cells. Insulin encourages the storage of glucose by fat and muscle cells to decrease the glucose in the blood, and tells the liver, which is the main site of glucose production, to make less glucose. After a meal, insulin encourages adipose cells to turn their glucose into fat, so if there is a large amount of glucose from a meal, this can encourage fat deposition.

Diabetes is another condition that we don't know the real prevalence of because it can be silently present for years before people get symptoms. There are multiple types of diabetes, usually grouped under the umbrella terms of "type 1" and "type 2." Type 1 is sometimes known as "juvenile diabetes," although it is possible to develop it at any age. Type 1 diabetes is an autoimmune disease, whereby the body decides that the beta islet cells of the pancreas that make insulin are actually the enemy and generates antibodies against them. People with type 1 diabetes don't make insulin and will rapidly die without insulin replacement.

The most common type of diabetes is type 2, and this is the one that can be silently going on in the background for years, not causing any evident symptoms until someone shows signs of organ damage. There are two aspects to developing type 2 diabetes. The first is the development of insulin resistance, so the pancreas has to work harder to keep blood glucose in the optimal range. When the pancreas can't keep up anymore, the person is said to have diabetes. While diabetes is associated with obesity, it's not clear whether obesity causes diabetes or whether they are associated conditions caused by the same underlying metabolic and inflammatory processes.

Diabetes is diagnosed when someone's blood sugar is greater than 7 mmol/liter (126 mg in 100 ml) while fasting, or a random blood glucose test shows a level greater than 11.1 mmol/liter (198 mg in 100 ml), or a measure of average blood glucose known as HbA1c is higher than 6.5 percent. People don't experience symptoms until the blood glucose rises to around 15 mmol/L because that is when glucose starts to be excreted by the kidneys, pulling water with it and causing polyuria, which then makes people extremely thirsty. The problem is that once this happens, people have often had high blood glucose for years. Every doctor has met the patient who proudly says they are completely healthy and haven't seen a doctor for years while the doctor is diagnosing kidney disease and heart failure caused by long-standing undiagnosed diabetes.

There are a few ways to screen for diabetes. All involve blood tests to check the blood glucose level and need to be organized by a doctor, usually a GP. There is no set age when diabetes screening should start; it varies depending on individual risk factors. People who have risk factors such as a family history of diabetes, being overweight, or women with a history of diabetes in pregnancy may need to start having screening at an earlier age. One of the reasons that this is important is that for some people lifestyle measures, like increased exercise and dietary changes, can reverse diabetes. For others, we have many very effective medications.

Brain hypometabolism and diabetes

Some people have referred to dementia as "type 3" diabetes. We know that people with diabetes are at high risk for getting dementia. Around 30 percent of people with type 2 diabetes have some cognitive impairment. People with poorly controlled diabetes or frequent episodes of hypoglycemia (low blood sugar) are at particular risk.

In the long term, diabetes can cause dementia in a couple of ways. People can develop damage in the large and small blood vessels, which can lead to the death of neurons, but insulin resistance itself means that the brain could effectively be "starving." As we noted in Question 3 about diagnosing dementia, it's possible to do a brain scan that measures glucose uptake in the brain to see which parts of the brain are active. The Alzheimer's Disease Neuroimaging Initiative, a study of 1,600 people ages fifty-five to ninety—some with normal cognition, some with mild cognitive impairment, and some with dementia—was started in 2003. People enrolled in the study underwent a range of testing, including brain imaging, and have been followed over time to look for things that predict dementia. The researchers looked at a subset of 159 people who also had type 2 diabetes. People with type 2 diabetes not only had lower brain volumes but they also had decreased metabolic activity in their brains, particularly in the frontal lobes and some of the sensory areas. Even for people on medications for diabetes with well controlled blood sugars, this association persisted, which means it is probably caused by the brain's inability to respond to glucose. Other studies have had similar findings.

How do I stop smoking?

When I think about my grandfather, I see him in a cloud of smoke, clutching his cigarettes in a gold package. My grandfather was a doctor, and like many doctors of his generation, he was a heavy smoker. He was diagnosed with dementia in his sixties. I have seen so much disease from smoking that I find it tragically sad to see people, especially young people, smoking. Early studies actually identified a lower risk for dementia with smoking, but a very nice analysis that looked at sources of funding showed that it was only studies that were funded by tobacco companies that showed smoking decreased the risk of dementia. In a review of nineteen studies looking at smoking and dementia, people who were current smokers compared to those who had never smoked were 1.27 times more likely to be diagnosed with dementia. People who smoked also had a greater yearly decline in cognitive function compared to nonsmokers.

In my social and family life, I don't know a single person who smokes. At work, I meet many. Smoking tends to track along socioeconomic lines, so people with lower incomes are more likely to have parents and friends who smoke and to be in an environment where it is socially normal to smoke. Australia has one of the lowest smoking rates in the world at 11.6 percent, which is half of what it was in 1991. We don't often see articles discouraging smoking in the lifestyle section of newspapers because it's not news that smoking is bad. The lifestyle section is also implicitly written for people with money, and most smokers have less than average spare cash, not least of which is because cigarettes are so expensive. Australia's success in reducing tobacco use is definitely worth celebrating, but it is important that we still support and encourage remaining smokers to give up and younger people to never start at all.

If you do smoke, I would strongly encourage you to go and see your primary care physician and ask about what support is available to stop smoking. As well as psychological support, there are also medications that can help.

Weight and cardiovascular health

Weight is a difficult topic to discuss. Obesity is a risk factor for dementia, and there is a lot about weight that is within our control. Part of our weight comes from genetics, but it is also connected to the food environment we are raised in. While your genes don't change in life, what does change is which genes are turned on or off: this is epigenetics. Epigenetics is influenced by the environment, including the environment you experienced as a fetus. If your mother didn't have enough to eat when she was pregnant with you, you probably have genes turned on to make sure your body is able to grab every available calorie—which can be a negative when you live in a world with an abundance of food. Gestational diabetes is also a risk factor for a child to have a higher risk of obesity in later life.

A major risk factor for obesity in Western societies is food insecurity. People with food insecurity, who can't be quite sure if they will have enough money for food tomorrow, do the rational thing and buy the cheapest food available. If you have hungry children, you know they will eat the supermarket chips and chicken nuggets, and with what budget you have you can get enough food on the table to fill tummies for around the same price as a large soy flat white at a fancy inner city café. We learn what to eat by what we eat as a family. As a parent I feel a big responsibility to my children to teach them to eat the right foods, including lots of vegetables, even though this is expensive and can result in throwing away uneaten food.

Highly processed food full of preservatives keeps longer and so makes more sense to buy for people on a low income. Paradoxically, those who spend the least on food are most likely to be obese.

It is worth remembering the lines that divide people into weight groups of "underweight," "healthy," "overweight," and "obese" were invented by humans, since we love to categorize things. Body mass index (BMI) is calculated as weight in kilograms divided by height in meters squared. It was originally devised by a mathematician. It is relatively easy to measure weight and height, but it is much harder to measure health behaviors, like using food and exercise recall diaries. People can still be overweight or obese and metabolically healthy. Some young male body builders, with lots of muscle and little fat, would be considered "overweight." It isn't as though risk increases exponentially when someone crosses from a weight in the overweight range to the obese range.

Nevertheless, there is some utility in measuring body mass index. At a population level, those at highest risk of death are those who have the lowest weight, as well as those with the highest weight. People with a body mass in the obese range also have an elevated risk for dementia.

The reasons behind the increased health risk of obesity are more complex than calories in and calories out. Body weight is also the result of hormonal changes, gut microbiome, and inflammation. Obesity is linked with higher levels of inflammation, and inflammation is linked with the development of dementia as discussed in Question 7, but it is also something of a chicken-and-egg situation, as it is not clear whether the obesity is driving inflammation, or the inflammation driving obesity.

For people with a very high weight-to-height ratio, there are also other conditions that can increase the risk of dementia. One is obstructive sleep apnea, where people's upper airway collapses as they fall into a heavy sleep, leading to multiple episodes of lack of oxygen at night. In a meta-analysis, people with sleep disordered breathing were around a third more likely to get dementia.

So . . . how to lose weight?

The secret reason the weight loss industry is so incredibly profitable is that they get a lot of return customers. People will go on a weight-loss program, have great success, then regain the weight. Let's face it, there wouldn't be so many books on the shelves about the perfect weight loss diet if one of them actually worked in the long term. Many different diets will produce weight loss, but it is keeping the weight off that is particularly difficult. For people who are suffering significant health problems related to weight, there are medical therapies to lose weight, such as meal replacement drinks, medications, or surgery.

For the majority of people, rather than encouraging weight loss per se, I think it is important to have a focus on quality nutrition, with nutrition considered as a gift to ourselves, something that we have because we deserve to feel great. Almost no one can live with severe restrictions for long periods of time, but as I will discuss in the next question, in the food environment we live in, it is important to understand how to make the best food choices for health.

The brain health checklist to discuss with your doctor

1. Get your blood pressure checked.

2. Get screened for diabetes.

3. Get your blood lipid profile checked (for cholesterol, etc).

4. Stop smoking.

5. Eat a brain healthy diet.

Are poverty and discrimination risk factors for dementia?

One of the most common myths about health is that everyone is equal. Dementia risk is profoundly unequal, starting from the time someone is born.

Louis-René Villermé was born in France in 1782, at a time when no one actually knew what caused most diseases. He studied surgery from 1801 to 1804, then he served in the Napoleonic Wars. After his service, he finished his thesis, then practiced medicine for four years before leaving to pursue research. While we think of scientific research discoveries in terms of laboratories, microscopes, and studying people with disease, I would argue that the scientific discoveries that have saved the most lives have been in the field of epidemiology. Epidemiology is the study of health and disease at the population level. Louis-René Villermé was the pioneer of social epidemiology—the study of the relationship between health and poverty. While his contemporaries were arguing whether disease was caused by contagion or environment, he was primarily concerned with what we now call "social determinants" of health.

Using population data from Paris, Villermé looked at the mortality rate, population density, and income. He was the first person to identify that people who were poor were more likely to die from disease.

This is one of the most important discoveries in science and medicine, and it's a discovery that is still sadly true to this day. Poverty makes people sick. It also causes dementia.

What does inequality have to do with dementia?

On my ward round, I have two patients who are living with dementia and are in the hospital, both with the same injury: a fractured hip. Doris's parents sent her to an expensive private school, and then her father was able to afford to send her to the university. Doris worked as a social worker, where she met her surgeon husband. They lived in a big house in an affluent suburb and sent their children to the same private schools they had attended themselves. Doris and her husband enjoyed a comfortable retirement, being prominent members at the golf club and enjoying annual overseas vacations.

Shirley lives with her daughter and grandchildren. Her father died when she was young, and her mother struggled to feed the children. Shirley had to work after school to help her mother pay the bills. She was often exhausted in school and struggled to learn.

Shirley left school at fourteen to work in a factory. Her husband liked to drink, and if Shirley didn't get between him and his pay check on a

Friday, the kids went hungry. Shirley's husband died of a heart attack when the kids were still young. She kept working until she had a back injury and was forced to stop. She also became immobile. Her pension didn't leave much left after paying the rent, so she had to buy whatever was on special at the supermarket, which was invariably ultra-processed food. The doctor she saw always rushed her in and out, so Shirley didn't really understand what she needed to do about her diabetes or all those pills for blood pressure and cholesterol. They were just one more expense.

Two women, both with dementia. The difference is that Shirley was diagnosed with dementia at seventy-three and Doris was diagnosed at ninety-two. Thanks to Doris's good start in life, she got almost twenty more years of brain health.

Socioeconomic status tends to be passed down through families, just like green eyes and a cleft chin. It influences all aspects of life and means that when it comes to brain health, two children born at the same time from different families can have very different risks of dementia from the start of life.

An uneven start to life

Dunedin is a university town in southern New Zealand. It is close to the Otago Peninsula, a famous wildlife haven with the only mainland albatross colony in the world.

Dunedin is also the site of a truly remarkable study that is helping us learn about the long-term impact of childhood disadvantage. Researchers recruited a group of 869 children who were born in 1972 and 1973, and have been assessing them regularly since they were three. The researchers were very careful to recruit children across a range of socioeconomic status (SES) groups. Over the years, the participants have had cognitive and health assessments.

From the very beginning, children whose parents had lower incomes had worse health and were more likely to have complications at birth. By the age of twenty-six, those in the low SES group had greater weight, higher waist–hip ratios, lower fitness, and poorer dental health, all of which are risks for dementia. It's also notable that this is in a country with universal healthcare. When this cohort was forty-five, they had MRI and an assessment of their cognitive function, which showed changes consistent with accelerated brain aging.

This group aren't yet in the age demographic where dementia is common, but in another study in Scotland that enrolled people born in 1936, researchers found that low socioeconomic status in childhood was associated with an increased risk of dementia and that people with a lower level of education had a more rapid trajectory of memory decline in older age.

For people with low SES as adults, the health disadvantages continue. SES continues to be associated with poorer health, including obesity and cardiovascular risk. People with low SES, measured as living in a deprived area and having low education and low-status, low-paying employment, have a 1.45 times higher risk of being diagnosed with dementia than those in the higher SES groups.

Inequality comes in many forms, and the reasons for low socioeconomic status are also many and varied. It is worth unpacking this further.

Brain health starts before conception

Before Darwin developed the theory of evolution, which so elegantly explains variation in species and change over time, another scientist had a different theory. Jean-Baptiste Lamarck was born in France in 1744, during the Enlightenment, when men (and women, who are largely forgotten by history) were trying to make scientific sense of the world. The first fossils were discovered in this time, and scientists became aware that the animals of the world had not always existed in their current form. Lamarck developed a theory that said characteristics acquired from the environment could be passed down from parent to offspring—for example, a blacksmith with a strong right arm having children with strong right arms. Lamarck's theory was discredited after the discovery of genes, but now with the discovery of epigenetics, we know that traits acquired though life can be passed down— though not in such obvious ways as big arm muscles. They are imparted in the genes that regulate our metabolism and immune function.

In September 1944, Dutch railway workers went on strike to try to stop the Nazis. They failed, and the Nazis responded by blocking food supplies. During the Dutch Hunger Winter, 20,000 people died of starvation. Women who were pregnant during this time were particularly vulnerable. In May 1945, the allied forces liberated the Netherlands, and nutrition returned to normal. This cohort of babies gestated during the famine, now older adults, provided an ideal natural experimental group. Compared to their siblings born after the war, this group was found more likely to be obese and have a higher risk of cardiovascular disease, diabetes, schizophrenia, and early death.

Our genes contain a set of instructions. Other than identical twins, we all have a different set of genes. Even identical twins, with their identical DNA, are not completely identical. They can be different heights, have different body weight, and develop different health conditions, but since they have the same genes, these differences are examples of epigenetics at work. Our genes are not always turned on: different genes will be switched on depending on various cell signals, and this can be influenced by the environment. Conditions occurring during a mother's pregnancy can influence which genes get turned on, and this continues through life. In the case of the Dutch babies gestated during the famine, genes got switched on that ensured those babies got as many calories as possible from their food, even though they were then born into a world where food shortage was no longer an issue. This turned out to be a disadvantage.

Increased cardiovascular risk is also bad for brain health. Around 4 to 10 percent of all women who are pregnant develop gestational diabetes. Children of mothers with gestational diabetes are more likely to develop diabetes themselves, although not the siblings born in pregnancies before the mother had diabetes. This suggests an epigenetic change. Babies of mothers with gestational diabetes can be exposed to excess sugar, which seems to trigger the metabolic "thrift" genes. These are the genes that make cells very good at extracting energy and lead to metabolic pathways linked with obesity and diabetes.

Diabetes and gestational diabetes are more common in low SES groups, so many children are starting life with a propensity for diabetes, which has serious long-term implications for brain health.

An enriched environment

For our brains to develop to their full potential we not only need optimal nutrition but also love and security. In the devastating studies of children raised in Romanian orphanages, where care was reduced to the absolute basics with almost no nurturing, it has been shown that these children often developed cognitive disabilities. Just living in poverty is enough for children to score lower on tests of cognitive abilities than their wealthier peers.

Our brains undergo incredible development in the first few years of life. A newborn baby can't control any of her limbs or speak, and she has no wants other than her need to be fed, cuddled, and warm. By the end of the first year, she may be walking, saying words, and getting very annoyed at her parents when they stop her from eating dirt. By the time a child is three, she can talk in sentences, run, play imaginary games, and have very big emotions (especially if you cut up her toast the wrong way!). This incredible brain development relies on an environment with loving caregivers who make her feel secure.

During brain development our neurons grow; they connect with one another, and the connections are pruned to make sure the most efficient brain circuitry is set up. Signals from the environment, such as loving parents, help this process.

Poverty has been simulated in animals. When juvenile rats are given limited nesting materials, in later life they have poorer memory. In rodents there is evidence that this is due to lack of maturation of brain circuits and lower levels of brain-derived neurotrophic factors—the messenger chemical that encourages brain cells to grow and connect.

Children are very receptive to the environment they live in. In a study of 1,099 children and adolescents in the United States, with an average age of eleven, children from low-income families showed structurally different brains on MRI scans at age eleven compared to children from well-off suburbs.

Middle-class parenting is very much about cultivation. Perhaps the difference is that when people are living in poverty the focus is on meeting needs? Most parents do their best, but a higher level of wealth means that the goalposts are different. It's not just food and shelter: it's music lessons, lots of books, and competition for the right preschool.

Education and dementia

Middle-class parenting is a competitive sport. Someone who had a good education knows it isn't just a good start in life; it unlocks doors that can provide a stable income for life. Education also provides skills for navigating the world and an ability to assess information, which can lead to making good health decisions later in life.

Studies worldwide have shown a relationship between lower levels of education and dementia. In one study of 593 people, individuals with less than eight years of education had 2.2 times higher risk of developing dementia than those with more years of education. Occupation also influences the risk of dementia: in a US cohort, those with low lifetime occupational attainment—meaning a low-status, low-income job—were at 2.25 times greater risk of developing dementia than those with high lifetime occupational attainment.

Education moderates the effect of Alzheimer's pathology. On average, people with higher levels of education have more damage to their brains before they get symptoms. This makes sense, since the diagnosis of Alzheimer's disease is based on being unable to function in day-to-day activities. If someone has more cognitive reserve to begin with, they will still be able to do these things even if they have lost some brain function. Brain reserve isn't just about the number of cells in the brain; it is also about how well connected they are to one another.

Even before school, in US studies it has been shown that around 40 percent of low-income parents never read to their children. Reading is a way to expose kids to a wider vocabulary of everyday words. It can also be a shared, loving time, which creates a love of books and motivation to read. This is one factor in kids from lower-income households having a less extensive vocabulary; so even before school there is a disadvantage.

During the COVID-19 pandemic, countries around the world conducted a social experiment with the closing of schools. The wealthy could access remote schooling, conducted online, relying on parents being able to afford devices and the Internet. This is likely to have compounded disadvantage and risks a generation of children from lower socioeconomic backgrounds being held back even more. While the people who make such policies are by and large highly educated and on high incomes, it will be low-income children who pay the long-term price. Curiously, closing schools in Melbourne actually had little impact on controlling the pandemic, according to an article whose authors included people who had instituted the policy.

Almost every parent does their best within their own circumstances to raise happy, healthy children. People who are wealthy learn the tricks of creating advantage for their children so they are ready to succeed in a world created by people like them. Every parent, and indeed every child, is not coming from the same start. There are additional factors, well beyond individual control, that contribute to dementia. Social structures that started generations ago persist today. Poverty is systemic.

What does poverty look like?

Poverty in developed countries like Australia and the United States can be relative or absolute. Absolute poverty includes people who are homeless. Relative poverty is those who are struggling. They have an unreliable income; they sometimes have enough to pay for food and rent, and sometimes don't. The people who fall into this group might be people who are on income support or those who do casual shift work.

Less money means fewer options. It can mean living far from work, which means lots of time in transit and little leisure time. It can mean living in a less comfortable suburb with little outdoor space. It can mean living in crowded housing where families are exposed to an increased risk of infections like COVID-19. Suburbs with poverty and rural areas have less access to primary care and allied health such as physiotherapists. Even for those who do not live below the poverty line, less money can mean making difficult decisions when it comes to health. Dentists are not covered by Medicare in Australia, so dental work can leave people thousands of dollars out of pocket. It is pretty easy to understand the links between poverty and poor dental health.

People living in poverty are also more likely to have psychiatric conditions, like depression and schizophrenia, although this may be a chicken-and-egg scenario, since these conditions can lead to disability and so fewer opportunities for work. Being poor can lead to high levels of stress, and being stressed worsens mental health. Poor mental health and low access to treatment means it is hard to work, and so the cycle perpetuates.

As mentioned in the previous Questions, poverty is also linked with obesity. The cheapest, most accessible foods are the ones with too many calories and very few nutrients. This means that if you have very few dollars to spend on food, the rational choice is whatever you can get cheaply, especially since these ultra-processed foods are designed to be very palatable. As noted elsewhere, this is why in countries like Australia, the UK, and the United States, food insecurity and poverty are linked with obesity.

People living on low incomes are also less physically active. It's not clear why this is. It may be due to fewer open spaces for walking and recreation.

Poverty also impacts health in other ways.

I remember reading a line in a book that stated that not everyone feels their health is a priority. As a naïve, middle-class twenty-something, that line was quite shocking because I, and many I know, make decisions based on "being healthy." Now, after almost two decades working in a public hospital, I see how this plays out. We all have a lot on our minds, and the mental space left over to make the choice to "do the right thing" is reduced when there is more stress in life. In a simple way, we have seen this in the COVID-19 pandemic, where during lockdown people who smoke started smoking more. The uncertainty and stress of a severe virus combined with social disconnection and financial worries meant that people fell into comforting habits.

When it comes to untangling the many threads that link the relationship between poverty, health behaviors, and dementia, a fundamental underlying truth is that people need to feel that they have the power to improve their health. They need to know that their behaviors matter, and they can make health a priority. This is a fundamental challenge of improving health at a population level.

Inequality is a killer

We like to pretend Australia is a classless society, but it is not. Australia has a serious inequality problem, and this is growing. People in the wealthiest quintile have a far lower risk of noncommunicable disease, which includes heart disease and diabetes, compared to those in the lowest quintile. People in the lowest quintile have around twice the risk of premature mortality. While Australia has one of the longest life expectancies in the world, prior to the pandemic, gains were slowing compared to other wealthy countries. Australia also has one of the highest rates of obesity in the world, and this is starting to translate to increased cardiovascular mortality in people under sixty-five. I worry we will soon cease to have rising life expectancy.

The risk factors for noncommunicable disease track along educational levels and income. This is why a child who is born into a family with loving parents who have stable housing and a good income, and who does well at school and goes on to attend university, is likely to live longer. This also translates to an unequal advantage in brain health.

The marshmallow test

There is a famous experiment called the marshmallow test. Three-year-olds were left alone in a room with a marshmallow and told that if they waited to eat it for fifteen minutes, they would get a second one. When these children were monitored in adolescence, it turned out that being able to hold out for that second marshmallow predicted academic and social success. Years later another group repeated the study, but this time the researchers collected more information about the children's families. These researchers found that the children who had developed the skill of delayed gratification as three-year-olds attained better academic results. But interestingly, they were also more likely to have mothers with university degrees and higher socioeconomic status. The lesson seems pretty clear: it is easier to delay gratification if you live in a stable and certain world.

The biomedical model, where a person develops symptoms, goes to the doctor for a diagnosis, and is given a cure, is deceptively simple. Disease, both communicable and noncommunicable, is driven hugely by underlying social factors that are easy to ignore and incredibly hard to fix. When health is framed as being a result of individual decisions, it automatically places blame on the sick. Personally, I find it incredibly upsetting that two children born in a rich country have a differing risk of dementia from the beginning of life.

Aboriginal and Torres Strait Islander people and dementia

I live on land that has been continuously occupied for around 60,000 years, and yet it would be unrecognizable to anyone who was here only two hundred years ago. The European invasion of Australia is such recent history that the effects still exist today. One effect is a significant gap in health outcomes.

In 2015 to 2017, life expectancy at birth for Aboriginal Australians was estimated to be 71.6 years for males and 75.6 years for females. In comparison, over the same period, life expectancy at birth for non-Indigenous Australians was 80.2 years for males and 83.4 years for females. Aboriginal people also have higher rates of dementia than the average Australian rates.

The Kimberley region of Australia is in remote Western Australia. The prevalence rates of dementia in Indigenous people of this region is around four to five times higher than the rest of Australia. The prevalence for people ages forty-five and older was 12.9 percent compared to 2.6 percent for the rest of Australia. Another study of Aboriginal people, ages forty to ninety-two, who live in an urban area, found that 21 percent had dementia compared to 6.8 percent of the Australian population in this age group.

The reasons for this are tied to the history of Australia and the violent beginnings of the country where I live.

A violent invasion

My ancestors were on the first boat to land in and invade Victoria, the state where I live. There is legal testimony from my ancestor about being attacked by the people who were already living here. This testimony echoes through the years as being written by a person trying to justify something inexcusable by denying the humanity of the local inhabitants. If your ancestors were white settlers from this time, chances are they took part in the violence as well or at least reaped the rewards of it.

The story of the invasion of Australia by white settlers is harrowing. Australia has 416 known sites where the European invaders massacred groups of Aboriginal people, including women and children. In parts of Australia, like Tasmania, the genocide was so extreme that people lost nearly all connection with the culture that had been an essential part of who they were. Lands were taken and cleared, fences and guns prevented movement, wetlands were drained, and sheep trampled over existing vegetation. Settlers brought all sorts of infectious diseases, such as tuberculosis, smallpox, and influenza.

My children are learning about this violent invasion in school, but when I was a child, I was taught that it was a peaceful settlement. We weren't taught about massacres, genocide, and slavery. We were taught history started with Captain Cook.

In Australia, Aboriginal and Torres Strait Islanders weren't even counted in the population until a referendum to change the constitution in 1967. There was also a formal government policy of removing children from their parents to take them to missions where they were prepared for a life of servitude. This happened from the 1800s to the 1970s and is referred to as the Stolen Generations. Children were denied access to culture and forbidden from speaking their language, which created intergenerational trauma that persists today. The history of slavery in the United States is well known, but Aboriginal people were also enslaved in Australia. To enslave someone is to fundamentally deny that they are human.

Even now, Aboriginal and Torres Strait Islander people face ongoing racism that impacts everyday life. In Australia, the rate of incarceration for non-Indigenous people is 166 per 100,000, but for Indigenous people it is 1,935 per 100,000. An example of why this happens is that in New South Wales between 2013 and 2017, 82.55 percent of all Indigenous people found with a non-indictable quantity of cannabis were pursued through the courts, compared with only 52.29 percent for the non-Indigenous population.

Medical racism

When I was at the university, we were taught that the reason Aboriginal people had such high rates of kidney disease was that they were born with fewer kidney cells. When I went back to look at the evidence for this, the statement was based on tiny studies that could in no way be generalized to explain the high kidney disease rate. Another thing we were taught was that Aboriginal people got diabetes because their metabolism was designed for a hunter-gatherer life of scarcity and couldn't cope with a Western diet, with the implication that Aboriginal people were less suited to modern life in an evolutionary sense.

At the time I accepted what my lecturer was saying. Now I look back and see that teaching medical students that Aboriginal people were less fit is teaching a form of eugenics.

Science is not cold hard facts; science is data and numbers generated by human beings, and without active efforts these cold hard facts can be subject to the racist interpretations of the very human scientists releasing the data.

The biomedical model of health is the model that dominates my working life. There is a lot about this model that works, such as that a person has a one-on-one interaction with another person who holds the health knowledge (me). I listen and then fit this description into a category of illness and prescribe a treatment. While I try to respect patient autonomy and the principle of shared decision-making, ultimately there is a huge imbalance of power. I am often in control of access to the treatment, and I am not sick. The biomedical model is also based on a Western model of health and medical research that has racist underpinnings, and for many Aboriginal people, this is a significant barrier to engaging with the health system. Risks for Aboriginal people range from poorer quality care, due to unconscious bias, to outright racism.

Inequitable access to health for people who are non-white has also been studied in other countries, notably the United States. At one hospital, a group of researchers identified that Black and Latinx people with heart failure were less likely to get admitted under cardiology for heart failure, instead going to general medicine, which meant a higher rate of readmission. By ignoring race, clinicians were actually letting their bias influence decision-making.

There is also evidence for these kinds of care gaps in Australia. In primary care, people who identify as Indigenous are less likely to have cardiovascular risk factors, such as blood pressure and diabetes screening, assessed compared to non-Indigenous people. This has important implications for dementia risk. In a 2016 study of Aboriginal people admitted to the hospital in South Australia with acute coronary syndrome, Aboriginal people were less likely to get an angiogram (dye into the heart to look for blocked vessels) than non-Aboriginal people. Interestingly, angiography was more likely if the person was accompanied by a family member or an Aboriginal liaison officer. In this study and others, Aboriginal people have been shown to be more likely to leave the hospital "against medical advice" (a problematic term), which is a troubling indication that white-dominant health institutions are not doing enough to communicate and engage with Indigenous patients.

Aboriginal communities have also been harmed by authorities claiming to do things for their own good. A distrust of institutions seems very reasonable in the context of the Stolen Generations and other atrocities.

One of the solutions to this has been the creation of the National Aboriginal Community Controlled Health Organisations (NACCHO). This provides national oversight to over 144 Aboriginal Community Controlled Health Organisations, which in turn provide primary care to around 410,000 people a year. NACCHO also advises and guides the Australian government on policy.

Of course, not all care—particularly complex acute care—can be provided in the community. This is where large organizations, like hospitals, also have a role in ensuring that the care is culturally safe.

How does all this cause dementia?

It's not just Aboriginal and Torres Strait Islander Australians who face health consequences of disadvantage and discrimination. Higher rates of dementia are found in many populations around the world who experience discrimination, including Black people in the United States and the UK.

Race is a social construct, but since human society follows such strict and complex social rules, it is still very real and has serious effects on health. Since the biological brain damage in dementia is so often the result of many social factors, it is not surprising that facing discrimination is part of this. In addition to the structural inequalities, the very experience of racism is associated with physiological stress.

The real cause of the health discrepancies between Aboriginal and non-Aboriginal Australians is because the white colonizers did everything they could to destroy a culture and shred families. The white colonizers did not succeed, and Australia is still home to the world's oldest civilization, but the consequences of this intergenerational trauma continue, along with the impact of racism today.

Since dementia is a life-course disease, influenced by early education, poverty, stress, and access to preventative healthcare, it is a perfect example of the fact that individual-level advice about lifestyle strategies is not enough. These things are important, but as a society we also need to care about everyone having the same access to education, adequate income, and housing. We need to consciously create a society that is free of discrimination and healthcare that is anti-racist.

Closing the gap

Uncle Terry Donovan, a Gumbaynggirr/Biripi man and researcher, says that Aboriginal people have the best culture in the world. He describes a beautiful culture of kinship, family, and community. From the time you are born into an Aboriginal family, you become the community's responsibility. In Aboriginal culture, elders are revered in a way other societies do not replicate. Sharing obligation means that everyone is looked after. Community looks after the health of the community.

Uncle Terry says that until Australia acknowledges its racist history, until we as a country act on racism in the here and now, we can't move forward. Truth-telling is key to reconciliation.

Working with people from a wide variety of backgrounds and life experiences, I have learned that people understand their own health needs. People want to be healthy, and they want their communities to be healthy. This isn't possible with a top-down approach. It needs to be a partnership between the people who administer the funds (government) and the people with the wisdom and understanding from the community. The idea of reconciliation is about strengthening all of Australia by strengthening relationships between Aboriginal and Torres Strait Islander peoples and non-Indigenous peoples.

The more I learn about Aboriginal and Torres Strait Islander concepts of health, the more I see how this is such an incredible strength. While the Western biomedical model is very focused on individuals, the lived reality is that health is a community concept. It's not enough for one person to get ahead; it has to be the community that is healthy together. Health is so much more than the physical: it includes culture and family connection. It is the idea that we all look after one another, from the elders to the young.

This isn't just relevant to decreasing chronic disease and dementia risk; this is relevant to recognizing that health is not just up to the individual, nor should it be. Health exists in community. This is particularly true for a life-course disease like dementia.

How do we address inequality?

Understanding health through an equality lens means considering gender, race, and disability, and how they intersect. It means integrating poverty, discrimination, and healthcare access as central when developing models of healthcare. There is a long way to go, but at least we have started the conversation.

QUESTION 20:

How do you avoid the stigma of living with dementia?

It was September 2020, and my colleagues and I sat on the lawn outside the hospital ward, a safe two meters apart, absolutely enraged by the morning's newspaper headline: "Shouting and kicking: Hospitals reveal new source of COVID spread."

We were outraged because the subjects of the headline were the patients we were looking after in the hospital, people who had caught COVID-19 at the hospital or in their nursing homes. The newspaper used a quote from a healthcare professional who was blaming "several distressed and delirious patients with COVID-19 [who] had been shouting, vocalizing loudly, and vigorously coughing," which was suspected to have started an outbreak affecting staff and patients. Around 60 percent of these patients also had dementia. People who could not speak up were blamed in a pattern I saw repeated around the world.

People with significant cognitive impairment are a terribly convenient scapegoat because they generally can't advocate for themselves and challenge a headline in a national newspaper. That the reporters unquestioningly accepted this explanation for the hospital outbreak shows how widespread stigma is around dementia. Put simply, it is hard to think of another group, including people with mental illness or an intellectual disability, who it would be acceptable to describe in such dehumanizing terms.

Dementia and stigma

At a webinar I attended, the presenter asked what the attendees thought of when they saw the word "dementia." The answers were almost all negative: fear, demise, uncertainty, loneliness, forgetfulness, brain illness, loss, uncertainty, stigma, grief, change of relationships, role change, people staying away, may be able to enjoy the moment more.

Surveys have shown that many people fear dementia more than any other disease, even cancer. In a survey commissioned by Dementia Australia, 94 percent of people living with dementia and 60 percent of caregivers have found themselves in an embarrassing situation due to dementia. People reported loneliness and disconnection. Almost half of the general public reported that they felt frustrated because they don't know how to help people with dementia.

Stigma comes from a place of fear and ignorance. We can only stigmatize someone if we "other" them. This stigma is also encouraged because people with dementia are so rarely visible in a public way.

People with dementia are hidden away

"Put your mask on! It's people like you who are making everyone sick! You selfish bastard; you don't care about anyone!"

The yelling cut through to Nina as she was trying to get her dog back on the leash after it chased a bird. She looked up and realized her dad was no longer right beside her; he had wandered off. Now he stood bewildered in the park as a stranger yelled at him for not obeying Melbourne's outdoor mask rule during the pandemic. Nina looked at the dog running dangerously close to the road, then looked at her scared father. She sprinted to her dad, grabbed his hand, and stood between him and the angry stranger.

"You don't understand; he has dementia."

There are standards of behavior in public, so we don't go to the supermarket in the nude or yell out in the middle of a movie. Part of improving care for people with dementia is creating more accessibility. It's impossible to look at someone and know whether they have dementia; it's an invisible disability. For someone who uses a wheelchair, it is obvious they need a ramp. For someone with an acquired, progressive intellectual disability like dementia, the first step is creating more understanding. Connection with other humans, especially those we don't know, comes from empathy. Being able to imagine ourselves in their position is key to this. Empathy also means setting aside judgment. The first step to creating a more dementia-accessible society is a better understanding of dementia to foster this empathy and tolerance.

Improving the understanding of dementia is also improving visibility.

Representations of dementia

"I'm Sebastien."

"I have a son called Sebastien."

"I'm your son."

On the video, she laughs in absolute delight, then they repeat the entire conversation.

One of the few places you can see representation of actual people with advanced dementia is TikTok, the social media app where people post short videos. The dementia hashtag has a huge 2.4 billion views. Some of the videos from healthcare professionals act out scenes to educate people on how to manage challenges in caring for people with dementia. Many of the videos are by caregivers, some showing beautiful moments, such as the woman who is delighted with her son; some show family caregivers how to connect with someone who doesn't recognize them using music or other activities.

Some videos are quite disturbing. In one I have seen, an elderly woman is looking for her little daughter. When the adult woman holding the camera says that she is her daughter, the expression in the elderly woman's eyes is baffled fear. Some videos are straight up mocking.

One of the problems with dementia care is that without representation, it is hard for the wider public, or even caregivers, to understand the condition. At the same time, while people with early dementia can consent to go on a TV show, I am going to assume that if someone doesn't recognize their own child, they don't have capacity to consent to a video of themselves on TikTok.

Maybe there is a place for caregivers to share videos of people with dementia if it will help other people, but would these people have wanted to be seen this way?

I think we also need to pick apart why it is seen as so humiliating to have cognitive disability. Perhaps the reason it is so hard to accept, why people wouldn't want others to see them this way, is that it makes us feel uncomfortable. Some of these videos show joy and love and the beauty of caregiving. Visibility can also teach others and make people feel less alone.

I don't think the answer to improved dementia awareness is to make people invisible. Respectful representation that highlights humanity, even for people with advanced dementia, is much more likely to lead to the change we need, like assisted living reform.

Dementia and institutionalization

In 1403, King Henry IV ordered a Royal Commission to investigate allegations of scandals, malpractice, and embezzlement of funds at the Bethlehem Hospital in London. Bethlehem Hospital was first created in 1247 as an institution funded by charity and taxes to house the poor and needy. It's not clear when it became an asylum for people with mental illness, but by 1403 there were records of people at Bethlehem with *mente capti*, or mental illness, as well as sick and elderly people. The long history of Bethlehem is punctuated by periodic external reviews, with people horrified at the conditions, attempts to improve things, followed by a long period when things fell back into disarray. For most of the institute's history, the warden responsible for the care of the inmates was also in control of finances. Many wardens took the opportunity to enrich themselves, while the vulnerable and chronically unwell residents suffered.

Reading the report from the aged care royal commission in Australia, which was published in 2021, it felt like nothing had changed. There was still neglect, and profit put before care. The assisted living sector relies on public funds to make a profit for providing care to some of the most vulnerable people in our society. Tax dollars go to these companies to the tune of around $60,000 per resident per year, amounting to hundreds of millions of dollars per year. Companies with a focus on profit have replaced the wardens of Bethlehem.

More than half of all people living in assisted living facilities have a diagnosis of dementia. In my experience of observing residents in assisted living, there are also a number who have dementia but haven't been given the diagnosis. This is relevant because people with dementia are particularly vulnerable to abuse if the dementia impacts their ability to remember and describe events or to communicate.

We no longer think that it is acceptable for people with long-term mental health disorders to live in institutions. Across Australia, many of these facilities have been closed and people moved to living in the community.

This was not without its own problems, since it was also used as a way to save the government money by not providing housing to people with long-term mental health problems.

One of the findings of the aged care royal commission was that it was not acceptable for young people with disabilities to live in assisted living facilities. In its own way, this finding could be interpreted as ageism. The facilities are acceptable for older people with disability but not younger people?

In an ideal world, care for older adults with cognitive disability would be provided in the community setting, or at least in small-group residential homes. Many people with moderate to advanced dementia do have high care needs, and these include personal care. Nursing homes are a convenient place to provide this. Many people with similar needs grouped together means it is possible to concentrate services.

The history of institutional care is one of compromising care for vulnerable people to make a profit. As noted previously, some companies are publicly listed; others are privately owned with complex corporate structures to minimize tax. Some of the families who own these are among the richest in Australia. This means people are becoming extremely wealthy while residents in assisted living get by on four dollars a day of food.

I firmly disagree with calls to put more public money in assisted living until there is reform and financial transparency. Without serious reform, care for people in nursing homes will always be at risk of coming second to profit.

John

John still remembers his first real kiss. Of course he had kissed Marjorie, the fiancée he found so easy to leave when he left Australia to do his PhD in Cambridge, but compared to his first real kiss, the kisses with Marjorie were about as exciting as tying his shoelaces.

The night of his real first kiss in Matthew's dormitory room, there was an unbearable anticipation while they sat not quite touching on the small couch. John barely dared to think that Matthew could feel this thing too, this forbidden thing. The moment when John was losing hope and said he better go, Matthew stepped forward and touched John's face, a question John answered by gently leaning forward to close the distance between them. The fire, the way it felt so right . . . he knew he never wanted it to stop.

The next morning, John left early but not early enough. He was seen. A rough night, he said, drank too much and passed out. John's double life of constant hiding had begun.

John wrote to Marjorie to end their engagement. He also tried to stop what he was doing. Everyone at Cambridge knew what had happened to Alan Turing. They all knew he was a criminal; they all knew about his shame. Each time, John and Matthew said this would be the last time, but it wasn't the last time until Matthew graduated and announced he was getting married.

John was heartbroken. He moved back to Sydney, taking a job as a college master at a university, a job he loved. But the job was also a trap. More than ever, he was constantly on guard, constantly aware that with the wrong look at someone he might lose his reputation and his job. He tried to set that part of his life aside, but he still found himself, every few weeks, at the toilet blocks in a suburb far from where he lived, looking for connection and release, hoping desperately that no one he knew would come his way, hoping more desperately that no one with a menacing glare and a cricket bat would come his way.

When John was thirty-eight, he met Tom, and they fell in love. Through Tom he found community and acceptance, and he had someone to come home to each night. Even if most of his family wanted nothing to do with John, he was happy beyond belief. The world was becoming more accepting, and homosexuality was no longer a crime. Then their friends started to die. Young men, wasting away. Tom and John cared for so many of their friends, who were again shunned and treated as less than human.

John and Tom survived, and grew together into old age until John nursed Tom through cancer.

John was alone again. His few friends who had survived the AIDS epidemic were also old and frail, and they found it hard to visit one another. John had lost touch with most of his family. All those years of hiding his secret life came back to him, and he didn't want anyone to visit him in his house. Once his dementia started, he became paranoid, those years of living with fear of discovery pressing on him. He became a recluse, even from the few friends and family he was still in touch with. One day he didn't answer his phone; his cousin called an ambulance, and they found John on the floor where he had fallen and been unable to get up.

John went to the hospital with a broken hip, and then to a nursing home. He still had a fear of other people, but the nursing home also had the dormitory rooms and structured days that felt familiar from his time in residential college. John's cousin had been very careful to choose a facility that had a policy of being LGBTQ-friendly, and asked the managers to do some education for their staff. Everyone at the facility was kind to John, and with his gentle grace and refined manners he was a great favorite with everyone at his new home.

Leave no one behind

John's story ends happily, but so many do not. If someone is already facing discrimination because of their race, gender, or sexual orientation, for example, the experience of this in the past and in present settings needs be considered, particularly formal care settings. For older adults who are LGBTQ, and have faced a life of discrimination, and even legal persecution, this may be a very important consideration, and especially for people living with HIV. HIV is something that the community needs to remain aware of, particularly in the assisted living setting as people living with HIV now reach old age.

Younger-onset dementia can cause more loss of years than older onset dementia, but it only accounts for 5 percent of all cases. Most people with dementia are old, and with that comes the additional stigma of agism. In some countries and cultures, memory loss is seen as a normal part of aging; this is especially true where people live with their extended family and can be supported. In a society like Australia, where independence is prized and many older adults live alone, the cognitive decline of dementia becomes a significant disability. This stigma can compound loneliness, especially if it leads to people avoiding the person living with dementia.

I'm not stupid

George

George knows he struggles to do new things. He knows that if he is out to dinner in a big group and everyone talks at once, he can have trouble following a conversation, and sometimes people exclude him. He notices that when he goes to the doctor, the doctor talks to his wife, not him. George knows that his mind has changed, but the one thing he wants people to know is that he is not stupid.

George loves when his grandchildren come to visit, especially when his granddaughter plays her violin for him and they connect over a shared love of music. His friend Paul picks him up every week to take him to the bowling club where they all know him so well. George loves these moments. He is connected; he is part of his community. He knows he can't do what he used to, but he is still valued.

One of the reasons dementia is so scary is that we live in a "hyper-cognitive society," to use a term coined by Stephen Post. We live in a society where people are valued for what they can produce and consume. Our society is one where individual achievement and independence are highly prized, even though humans are, by our very nature, interconnected and dependent on one another. We have created a false construct in modern society where we have the illusion that we are able to get by alone and independent when it is the work of procuring what we need that has been invisibly outsourced. For most of human history we lived in interconnected family groups where everyone had a role in helping others and in getting the necessities of life; now we live in small households where our water comes in pipes, heat turns on with the flick of a switch, and we never see the work of growing and collecting the food we purchase at the supermarket. This fuels the myth of independence that we cling to as an identity. Dementia rips holes in that myth and shows how dependent we actually are.

When people have dementia, especially advanced dementia, community and care are more important than ever. People living with dementia matter, their contributions to society, friends, and family matter. Despite general societal attitudes, needing help does not make someone a less valuable human.

Sometimes we come across ideas that are uncomfortable, things that make us feel bad. It is far too easy to avoid them, but if we don't sit with the discomfort, we don't grow. If reading about dementia, the idea of getting dementia, or being a caregiver for someone with dementia has made you uncomfortable, you need to ask yourself why. If you find your own negative ideas, it's time to learn more about dementia and about yourself.

How do we live well with dementia?

The first thing Frances does when she gets up is make herself a coffee. She presses a button, and the warm milky coffee is ready to go. Some days she remembers to make toast as well. An efficient, clear voice with a friendly tone calls out, "Time to take your medicine, Frances." This voice will remind her three times to walk over to her medication box, where the compartment for the right time and day is open. Once Frances has taken her medications, the reminder will stop. The doorbell rings, and Leah is there. She greets Frances with a big smile. Leah or Joan come every day; Frances has gotten to know them well. Leah asks Frances if she would like her to stay outside the bathroom while she showers, just in case. Frances likes knowing she is there, as she does worry about falling. Leah checks the fridge and uses her phone to order more groceries.

After Frances is showered and dressed, Leah says goodbye to her. Shortly afterward a bus comes. The driver is friendly and familiar. "Hello, Frances.

Would you like to come to music? Today, they are writing a song." Before she retired, Frances was a music teacher, so she helps to run the class. Everyone loves it. They all have a good laugh. While she is there, Frances also has a great meal. She has a second serve and dessert.

After she gets home, Frances goes for a walk. At one point she is unsure where she is, but everyone recognizes her, and someone always helps her. Her watch can detect sudden sharp movements toward the ground and has a GPS, so if she falls, someone will be alerted to look for her. After she gets home, her daughter gives her a call. They have a wonderful discussion about the grandchildren and reminisce about when her daughter was young. Frances's daughter tells her that tomorrow she will work from home at Frances's house. Frances might remember this, or it might be a lovely surprise when her daughter turns up.

Frances has some fruit and yoghurt for dinner. She goes to sleep happy, and while she can't remember the details of all she did, she is left with a feeling of contentment.

The dignity of risk

Frances's day is quite a normal day, but it is a good day. It is a day someone lives with dementia, perhaps a little imperfectly, but independently and using her skills. She is someone who is supported with technology to be independent. She lives in a community where people recognize her and help her, where the community understands what dementia is and they value and respect all residents.

Frances does not live a perfectly safe life. Sometimes she forgets breakfast or her medications. Sometimes she just has a banana for dinner. She had a fall last year and could have another, but here is a thought you must sit with: none of us live lives of perfect safety. Such a thing does not exist.

Living well with dementia means accepting the dignity of risk. Many people with dementia will be able to live independent lives, but they may not be perfectly safe. People with dementia can forget to eat, for example, or have difficulty preparing a meal, but there are ways to ensure they are still getting adequate nutrition. Sometimes this can be making sure that people get one really good meal per day and providing high-caloric snacks clearly visible around the house. This approach to dementia care is less restrictive than having someone move into assisted living.

Is technology the answer?

The safety issue does also bring up some ethical dilemmas. My husband and I have location sharing on our phones. We have an agreement that we can track each other. Frances wears a watch that allows people to track her and to be aware if she falls. Did she consent to this? How does she feel about it? Even if she is not aware, is this justified because it helps her family to support her staying at home?

There are even more intrusive options in home monitoring, such as sensors that monitor a person's movements around the house and whether or not they are opening a fridge. One of these is combined with a care robot that looks like a vase with fake flowers and eyes. A cheery video promises that if the sensor sees someone not moving at mealtime, it will prompt them to get a meal. To be honest, the talking vase robot hybrid is a little disturbing, and I am not really sure that many people living with dementia will respond well to one telling them to eat.

There are also other potential uses, like programming a device to prompt the person when they have an appointment and to automatically call a taxi.

For people who already have some sort of virtual home assistant, such as those of Google or Amazon, it is not such a stretch to imagine it could start to take on more of a guidance role. Of course, there would need to be careful controls in place so it didn't prompt the person with dementia to start buying things.

These technologies are a form of surveillance, but they do have potential to help in the balance of ensuring that someone is able to maintain their independence longer. I do have patients who strongly want to live at home, but they are unable to problem solve things like how to call an ambulance or even how to press an alarm on a pendant. Technology might be the answer.

Routine and memory

One of the most protective factors is also one of the most mundane: routine. The majority of my work is in the hospital setting. The hospital setting is incredible for providing efficient medical intervention, but it is not usually good for people with dementia. Not only do we keep people awake at night and serve them unappealing food, but being in the hospital also takes people out of their routine. This is sometimes the first time it becomes apparent someone has dementia. Short-term memory loss in the home, which wasn't causing any major problems in the familiar environment with family supports, is unmasked as dementia.

When someone doesn't have as much ability to plan and problem solve, routine and familiarity are important protective factors. Things like keeping to the usual time of day that someone bathes and eats are important in their care at all stages of dementia. If someone spent their life working as a garbage collector, rising extremely early to go and be physically active, this can be important to include in their care.

Imagine if, like a diabetes educator, there was a dementia educator. Someone whom the person with dementia and their loved ones could check in with to help them link to services and activities. There are day programs available for people to engage in activities they enjoy and socialize, but these are few and far between.

What works?

When someone gets a label of dementia, there can be a perception that they have lost their skills, but our brain is not so linear as all that. Different memories and abilities are stored in different ways and can remain.

One of the challenges in dealing with dementia is that there is just not enough research into the right supports for people, nor into what living well with dementia looks like.

In the UK, everyone with dementia gets to attend fourteen sessions of group cognitive stimulation therapy. This therapy focuses on mental stimulation in a fun environment with an emphasis on inclusion and connection.

The other advantage to this is it gives people with dementia and their caregivers the chance to meet other people sharing the experience. Not everyone with dementia will want to spend time with other people with dementia, but for some it can be helpful to share the experience with those who understand.

In Australia, people can access support groups through the organization Dementia Australia, but there is still a real lack of public funding within the health system for ongoing support.

The future is now

Almost every week there is a headline about a new cure for dementia. Invariably, it is in mice. None of these are yet to translate to real improvements in humans. Yet dementia is here now. In countries such as the UK, Australia, and the United States, we are in a demographic shift so slow that we haven't noticed what a completely remarkable time we are living in. We are in the first era where most people are expected to live to old age. This is absolutely unprecedented. To put it in perspective, in 1901 the average life expectancy for a male in Australia was 55 and for a female it was 59. It was common for children to die in their first years of life. Now, the average life expectancy is 82.9.

Dementia is an age-related condition. When there are more older people, there will be more people with dementia. One really important positive caveat to this is that the risk of dementia is actually decreasing with better management of cardiovascular risk factors, such as high blood pressure, and with higher levels of education. Nevertheless, more older people does mean more people in the age group where rates of dementia start to rise.

The opposite of a good life

For many people with dementia, the years of the pandemic were the opposite of living well with dementia. People with dementia are at a higher risk of bad outcomes with COVID-19. The years of isolation also caused harm. As early as 2020, there were 13,000 additional deaths in people with dementia from non-virus causes between March and June in the UK, although some of these deaths were likely from COVID due to limited testing at that time. In Australia, in the first half of 2022, deaths from dementia were 20 percent above baseline, but this trend had already started in the first half of 2021 when Australia was COVID-free, so we can't fall back on simply blaming one virus.

A review of the impact of lockdown on people living with dementia found that people experienced worsening of cognition, behavioral and psychological symptoms, and a decline in their level of function. Worryingly there was also an increase in the prescription of antipsychotics and benzodiazepines.

As a hospital-based geriatrician, I have looked after people who died from COVID-19, so I take this disease seriously, but I also take the decline and deaths of people living with dementia from non-COVID-19 causes just as seriously. As a terminal condition, deaths from dementia cannot be completely prevented, but I have seen people who have had a major decline, such as significant weight loss, because family couldn't come over to help them eat during lockdowns in residential care. That absolutely contributed to their earlier death.

Other people became too scared to go outside and do activities such as lawn bowling. One of the key, avoidable mistakes in the pandemic was the disproportionate focus on policing outdoor spaces, when this could have been a key strategy to help people stay active and get the cognitive stimulation from being with others that is an essential component of health.

The lesson from the pandemic years is that personal connection and care are absolutely nonnegotiable for health.

I live in Melbourne, where our government's response to the pandemic was primarily to impose harsh social restrictions, which were heavily policed. I grieved for the patients I cared for who died, but I also grieved for what was lost, and the groups who lost the most were children and the very elderly. The very elderly, who declined when they lost their routines, care packages, socialization and opportunities for connection, will never get this back.

Going forward, we can never again lose sight that these are critical, nonnegotiable aspects of living well with dementia.

The goals of dementia care

One of my favorite questions to ask my patients is what they like to do. This can lead us to a discussion about what is important to them and to work on person-centered goals. Speaking with patients about this and developing a care partnership is where individual health intersects with the medical system. Perfect health is not a meaningful goal because, no matter what, it all ends the same way. What is meaningful is connection, joy, and feeling part of something bigger than yourself—the sense that life has meaning.

The big-picture goals of dementia care also need to be put in the context of day-to-day life. We spend a lot of our time doing things we enjoy, but this differs for all of us. Some people like sports, some people like the theater, some people enjoy art, and others like to garden. Food choices are another example. People have different preferences and even different times of day when they prefer to take their meals. Either way, life is to be lived.

Similarly, living well looks different to everyone, but for many people it means retaining independence and maintaining function. As I hope I have made clear throughout this book, it is also about joy, connection, and fun. It is entirely possible that one day I will be a very old woman who does not recognize my family. This prospect is devastating, but maybe I would not be unhappy. Maybe someone would give me a doll that takes me back to the incredible moment I first held my children as newborns, thereby gifting my children the view of me holding them when they were babies.

There are risks in putting off what we really want to do in life, whether it is travel, getting that job, or learning a musical instrument. Life is not about the destination, it is about enjoying the process along the way.

The price of the very long life that I want is that I will age and might get dementia, but it is a price I am willing to pay for all the wonder that comes from being alive.

Acknowledgments

One of the best things about writing a book is having the opportunity to reach out to experts I admire across the world (and some closer to home) and ask them to donate their time so I can ask all sorts of questions. All these very busy people responded with such generosity to help me understand dementia: Professor Robert Howard, Professor Shaun O'Keeffe, Professor Jason Karlawish, Professor Turhan Kanli, Professor Muireann Irish, Professor Kwang Lim, Professor Sharon Goldfield, Uncle Terrence Donovan, Dr. Kylie Radford, Ellen Finlay, Dr. Madeleine Healey, Associate Professor Rosie Watson, Associate Professor Samantha Loi, Maree McCabe AM, Dr. Marita Long, Dr. Leonie Simpson, and Associate Professor Kate Laver.

The caregivers I spoke to shared some of the most profound experiences of their lives. I know for some it was incredibly hard, and I want you to know that hearing your stories has helped make me a better doctor. I want to thank Anne Fairhall, Jo Hallinan, Fiona McKay, and Kate. I also want to thank all the people who informally shared their stories with me when I told them that I was writing a book about dementia.

Writing involves a lot of time sitting alone, getting words on a page, then worrying about whether those words are any good. Unlike in book one, this time I had my incredibly supportive writing group to talk craft and read early drafts. I want to thank Dr. Neela Janakiramanan, Dr. Mariam Tokhi, Dr. Stephanie Convery, and Isy Oderberg (who is practically a doctor as well).

I would like to thank my agent, Margaret Gee, who came up with the idea of framing the book around questions, which was really when the book concept gelled for me!

Thank you to Rebecca Wylie for your thoughtful edit.

I could not have asked for better editorial support than the team at HarperCollins. Thank you to Shannon Kelly and Mary Rennie. Mary, all the work you did helped me to make the message in this book so much clearer and really helped me to refine the complex ideas I was trying to express.

I want to thank my three children, Lily, Harvey, and Arthur, for their patience while I stole time away on mornings and weekends to write. I love you all so much.

Last, and most important, I could not have written this book without the support of my husband, Michael, both the practical support and the emotional support for all the times it felt too hard. Thank you for everything you do for our family.

Resources

Dementia Australia has help and information sheets and provides education resources, both online and in support groups, www.dementia.org.au.

NHS
The UK NHS has information for people who want to learn more about dementia, https://www.nhs.uk/conditions/dementia/about/.

The US National Institute of Aging has a range of factsheets about dementia, https://www.nia.nih.gov/health/topics/dementia.

Introduction
Dementia Language Guidelines, Dementia Australia, 2021.

Question 1: What is dementia and are you at risk?
American College of Medical Genetics/American Society of Human Genetics Working Group on ApoE and Alzheimer Disease, "Statement on Use of Apolipoprotein E Testing for Alzheimer Disease," *Jama*, 1995; 274(20): 1627–1629.

Australian Institute of Health and Welfare, *Dementia in Australia*, 2022.

Evans, DA, et al., "Incidence of Alzheimer Disease in a Biracial Urban Community: Relation to Apolipoprotein E Allele Status," *Archives of Neurology*, 2003; 60(2): 185–189.

Farias, ST, et al., "Progression of Mild Cognitive Impairment to Dementia in Clinic vs Community-Based Cohorts," *Archives of Neurology,* 2009; 66(9): 1151–1157.

Force, UPST, "Screening for Cognitive Impairment in Older Adults: US Preventive Services Task Force Recommendation Statement," *JAMA,* 2020; 323(8): 757–763.

Jansen, WJ, et al., "Prevalence of Cerebral Amyloid Pathology in Persons Without Dementia: A Meta-Analysis," *JAMA,* 2015; 313(19): 1924–1938.

Rooney, MR, et al., "Risk of Progression to Diabetes Among Older Adults with Prediabetes," *JAMA Internal Medicine,* 2021; 181(4): 511–519.

Ryman, DC, et al., "Symptom Onset in Autosomal Dominant Alzheimer Disease: A Systematic Review and Meta-Analysis," *Neurology,* 2014; 83(3): 253–260.

Wilson, RS, et al., "Vulnerability to Stress, Anxiety, and Development of Dementia in Old Age," *Am J Geriatr Psychiatry,* 2011; 19(4): 327–334.

Zallen, DT, "'Well, Good Luck with That': Reactions to Learning of Increased Genetic Risk for Alzheimer Disease," *Genetics in Medicine,* 2018; 20(11): 1462–1467.

Question 2: What are the symptoms of dementia?

Budson, AE, and BH Price, "Memory Dysfunction," *New England Journal of Medicine,* 2005; 352(7): 692–699.

Cooper, C, et al., "The Meaning of Reporting Forgetfulness: A Cross-Sectional Study of Adults in the English 2007 Adult Psychiatric Morbidity Survey," *Age and Ageing,* 2011; 40(6): 711–717.

Jäkel, S, and L Dimou, "Glial Cells and Their Function in the Adult Brain: A Journey Through the History of Their Ablation," *Frontiers in Cellular Neuroscience,* 2017.

Liesinger et al., "Sex and Age Interact to Determine Clinicopathologic Differences in Alzheimer's Disease," *Acta Neuropathol,* 2018; 136(6): 873–885.

Mitchell, AJ, et al., "Risk of Dementia and Mild Cognitive Impairment in Older People with Subjective Memory Complaints: Meta-Analysis," *Acta Psychiatr Scand*, 2014; 130(6): 439–451.

Oxford Textbook of Cognitive Neurology and Dementia, Oxford University Press, 2019.

Pisani, MA, et al., "Days of Delirium Are Associated with 1-Year Mortality in an Older Intensive Care Unit Population," *Am J Respir Crit Care Med*, 2009; 180(11): 1092–1097.

Rahman, A, et al., "Sex and Gender Driven Modifiers of Alzheimer's: The Role for Estrogenic Control Across Age, Race, Medical and Lifestyle Risks," *Frontiers in Aging Neuroscience*, 2019; 11: 315.

Tsui, A, et al., "The Effect of Baseline Cognition and Delirium on Long-Term Cognitive Impairment and Mortality: A Prospective Population-Based Study," *The Lancet Healthy Longevity*.

Unkenstein, AE, et al, "Understanding Women's Experience of Memory over the Menopausal Transition: Subjective and Objective Memory in Pre-, Peri-, and Postmenopausal Women," *Menopause*, 2016; 23(12): 1319–1329.

Question 4: What are the types of dementia?
Kavirajan, H, and LS Schneider, "Efficacy and Adverse Effects of Cholinesterase Inhibitors and Memantine in Vascular Dementia: A Meta-Analysis of Randomised Controlled Trials," *Lancet Neurol*, 2007; 6(9): 782–792.

Rolinski, M, et al., "Cholinesterase Inhibitors for Dementia with Lewy Bodies, Parkinson's Disease Dementia and Cognitive Impairment in Parkinson's Disease," *Cochrane Database Syst Rev*, 2012(3).

Takeda, A, et al., "A Systematic Review of the Clinical Effectiveness of Donepezil, Rivastigmine and Galantamine on Cognition, Quality of Life and Adverse Events in Alzheimer's Disease," *Int J Geriatr Psychiatry*, 2006; 21(1): 17–28.

Question 5: Do we actually know what causes Alzheimer's?

Ayton, S, et al., "Brain Iron Is Associated with Accelerated Cognitive Decline in People with Alzheimer Pathology," *Molecular Psychiatry*, 2020; 25(11): 2932–2941.

Bejanin, A, et al., "Tau Pathology and Neurodegeneration Contribute to Cognitive Impairment in Alzheimer's Disease," *Brain*, 2017; 140(12): 3286–3300.

Glenner, GG, and CW Wong, "Alzheimer's Disease: Initial Report of the Purification and Characterization of a Novel Cerebrovascular Amyloid Protein," *Biochem Biophys Res Commun*, 1984; 120(3): 885–890.

Iacono, D, WR Markesbery, M Gross, et al., "The Nun Study: Clinically Silent AD, Neuronal Hypertrophy and Linguistic Skills in Early Life," *Neurology*, 2009; 73(9): 665–673.

King, A, "The Search for Better Animal Models of Alzheimer's Disease," *Nature*, 2018; 559(7715): 13–15.

Kyle, RA, "Amyloidosis: A Convoluted Story," *Br J Haematol*, 2001; 114(3): 529–538.

Makin, S, "The Amyloid Hypothesis on Trial," *Nature Outlook*, 2018.

Masters, CL, et al., "Amyloid Plaque Core Protein in Alzheimer Disease and Down Syndrome," *Proceedings of the National Academy of Sciences*, 1985; 82(12): 4245–4249.

Maurer, K, S Volk, and H Gerbaldo, "Auguste D and Alzheimer's Disease," *The Lancet*, 1997; 349(9064): 1546–1549.

Messerli, FH, "Chocolate Consumption, Cognitive Function and Nobel Laureates," *New England Journal of Medicine*, 2012; 367(16): 1562–1564.

Müller, UC, T Deller, and M Korte, "Not Just Amyloid: Physiological Functions of the Amyloid Precursor Protein Family," *Nature Reviews Neuroscience*, 2017; 18(5): 281–298.

Oyama, F, et al., "Down's Syndrome: Up-Regulation of Beta-Amyloid Protein Precursor and Tau mRNAs and Their Defective Coordination," *J Neurochem*, 1994; 62(3): 1062–1066.

Pietrzak, RH, et al., "Trajectories of Memory Decline in Preclinical Alzheimer's Disease: Results from the Australian Imaging, Biomarkers and Lifestyle Flagship Study of Ageing," *Neurobiol Aging*, 2015; 36(3): 1231–1238.

Popper, KR, *Objective Knowledge: An Evolutionary Approach*, Clarendon Press, 1972.

Saez-Atienzar, S, and E Masliah, "Cellular Senescence and Alzheimer Disease: The Egg and the Chicken Scenario," *Nature Reviews Neuroscience*, 2020; 21(8): 433–444.

Tanzi, RE, and L Bertram, "Twenty Years of the Alzheimer's Disease Amyloid Hypothesis: A Genetic Perspective," *Cell*, 2005; 120(4): 545–555.

Question 6: What is the role of aging in dementia?

Bernhardt, L, and CA Lawson, "Early Menopause and Risk of Cardiovascular Disease: An Issue for Young Women," *The Lancet Public Health*, 2019; 4(11): 539–540.

Bonfanti, L, and I Amrein, "Editorial: Adult Neurogenesis: Beyond Rats and Mice," *Front Neurosci*, 2018; 12: 904.

de Magalhaes, JP, and JF Passos, "Stress, Cell Senescence and Organismal Ageing," *Mech Ageing Dev*, 2017.

Franceschi, C, et al., "Inflammaging: A New Immune–Metabolic Viewpoint for Age-Related Diseases," *Nature Reviews Endocrinology*, 2018; 14(10): 576–590.

Larson, EB, et al., "New Insights into the Dementia Epidemic," *N Engl J Med*, 2013; 369(24): 2275–2277.

López-Otín, C, et al., "The Hallmarks of Aging," *Cell*, 2013; 153(6): 1194–1217.

Manson, JE, and TK Woodruff, "Reproductive Health as a Marker of Subsequent Cardiovascular Disease: The Role of Estrogen," *JAMA Cardiology*, 2016; 1(7): 776–777.

Prince, M, et al., "The Global Prevalence of Dementia: A Systematic Review and Metaanalysis," *Alzheimers Dement*, 2013; 9(1): 63–75e62.

Saez-Atienzar, S, and E Masliah, "Cellular Senescence and Alzheimer
   Disease: The Egg and the Chicken Scenario," *Nature Reviews
   Neuroscience*, 2020; 21(8): 433–444.

Zhu, D, et al., "Relationships Between Intensity, Duration, Cumulative
   Dose, and Timing of Smoking with Age at Menopause: A Pooled
   Analysis of Individual Data from 17 Observational Studies," *PLoS Med*,
   2018; 15(11): e1002704.

Question 7: Does inflammation cause dementia?

Bachiller, S, et al., "Microglia in Neurological Diseases: A Road Map
   to Brain-Disease Dependent-Inflammatory Response," *Frontiers in
   Cellular Neuroscience*, 2018; 12(488).

Forrester, JV, PG McMenamin, and SJ Dando, "CNS Infection and
   Immune Privilege," *Nature Reviews Neuroscience*, 2018; 19(11): 655–671.

Franceschi, C, et al., "Inflammaging: A New Immune–Metabolic
   Viewpoint for Age-Related Diseases," *Nature Reviews Endocrinology*,
   2018; 14(10): 576–590.

Hampshire, A, et al., "Cognitive Deficits in People Who Have Recovered
   from COVID-19," *EClinicalMedicine*, 2021; 39.

Holmes, C, et al., "Systemic Inflammation and Disease Progression
   in Alzheimer Disease," *Neurology*, 2009; 73(10): 768–774.

Johnston, RB, "An Overview of the Innate Immune System," *UpToDate*,
   March 5, 2021.

Lövheim, H, et al., "Herpes Simplex Infection and the Risk of Alzheimer's
   Disease: A Nested Case-Control Study." *Alzheimers Dement*, 2015; 11(6):
   587–592.

Pandharipande, PP, et al., "Long-Term Cognitive Impairment After Critical
   Illness," *New England Journal of Medicine*, 2013; 369(14): 1306–1316.

Pasqualetti, G, DJ Brooks, and P Edison, "The Role of Neuroinflammation
   in Dementias," *Current Neurology and Neuroscience Reports*, 2015;
   15(4): 17.

Tzeng, NS, et al., "Anti-Herpetic Medications and Reduced Risk of Dementia in Patients with Herpes Simplex Virus Infections: A Nationwide, Population-Based Cohort Study in Taiwan," *Neurotherapeutics*, 2018; 15(2): 417–429.

Xu, E, et al., "Long-Term Neurologic Outcomes of COVID-19," *Nature Medicine*, 2022; 28(11): 2406–2415.

Question 8: Does dementia begin in the gut?

"Australia and New Zealand Ban European Beef," *The Guardian*, January 6, 2001.

Bichell, RE, "When People Ate People, a Strange Disease Emerged," NPR. org, September 6, 2016.

Call, ME, "Antigen-Presenting Cells," *UpToDate*, February 22, 2022.

Chelakkot, C, J Ghim, and SH Ryu, "Mechanisms Regulating Intestinal Barrier Integrity and Its Pathological Implications," *Experimental & Molecular Medicine*, 2018; 50(8): 1–9.

Furness, JB, "The enteric nervous system and neurogastroenterology," *Nature Reviews Gastroenterology & Hepatology*, 2012; 9(5): 286–294.

Gao, X, et al., "A Prospective Study of Bowel Movement Frequency and Risk of Parkinson's Disease," *Am J Epidemiol*, 2011; 174(5): 546–551.

Govindarajan, N, et al., "Sodium Butyrate Improves Memory Function in an Alzheimer's Disease Mouse Model when Administered at an Advanced Stage of Disease Progression," *J Alzheimers Dis*, 2011; 26(1): 187–197.

Ho, L, et al., "Protective Roles of Intestinal Microbiota Derived Short Chain Fatty Acids in Alzheimer's Disease-Type Beta-Amyloid Neuropathological Mechanisms," *Expert Review of Neurotherapeutics*, 2018; 18(1): 83–90.

Houser, MC, and MG Tansey, "The Gut–Brain Axis: Is Intestinal Inflammation a Silent Driver of Parkinson's Disease Pathogenesis?," *NPJ Parkinson's Disease*, 2017; 3(1): 3.

Kresl, P, et al., "Accumulation of Prion Protein in the Vagus Nerve in Creutzfeldt–Jakob Disease," *Ann Neurol*, 2019; 85(5): 782–787.

Madore, C, et al., "Microglia, Lifestyle Stress, and Neurodegeneration," *Immunity*, 2020; 52(2): 222–240.

Saji, N, et al., "Analysis of the Relationship Between the Gut Microbiome and Dementia: A Cross-Sectional Study Conducted in Japan," *Scientific Reports*, 2019; 9(1): 1008.

Saji, N, et al., "Relationship Between Dementia and Gut Microbiome-Associated Metabolites: A Cross-Sectional Study in Japan," *Scientific Reports*, 2020; 10(1): 8088.

Terry, N, and KG Margolis, "Serotonergic Mechanisms Regulating the GI Tract: Experimental Evidence and Therapeutic Relevance," *Handb Exp Pharmacol*, 2017; 239: 319–342.

Valles-Colomer, M, et al., "The Neuroactive Potential of the Human Gut Microbiota in Quality of Life and Depression," *Nature Microbiology*, 2019.

Winge, K, D Rasmussen, and LM Werdelin, "Constipation in Neurological Diseases," *J Neurol Neurosurg Psychiatry*, 2003; 74(1): 13–19.

Zhang, B, et al., "Inflammatory Bowel Disease Is Associated with Higher Dementia Risk: A Nationwide Longitudinal Study," *Gut*, 2021; 70(1): 85–91.

Question 9: Does stress cause dementia?

Aschbacher, K, et al., "Maintenance of a Positive Outlook During Acute Stress Protects Against Pro-Inflammatory Reactivity and Future Depressive Symptoms," *Brain Behav Immun*, 2012; 26(2): 346–352.

Barnes, DE, et al., "Midlife vs Late-Life Depressive Symptoms and Risk of Dementia: Differential Effects for Alzheimer Disease and Vascular Dementia," *Arch Gen Psychiatry*, 2012; 69(5): 493–498.

Chen, H, M Lombès, and D Le Menuet, "Glucocorticoid Receptor Represses Brain-Derived Neurotrophic Factor Expression in Neuron-Like Cells," *Mol Brain*, 2017; 10(1): 12.

Friedman, M, et al., "Cognitive and Neural Mechanisms of the Accelerated Aging Phenotype in PTSD," *American Journal of Geriatric Psychiatry*, 2019; 27(3S): S203.

Günak, MM, et al., "Post-Traumatic Stress Disorder as a Risk Factor for Dementia: Systematic Review and Meta-Analysis," *British Journal of Psychiatry*, 2020; 217(5): 600–608.

MacQueen, G, and T Frodl, "The Hippocampus in Major Depression: Evidence for the Convergence of the Bench and Bedside in Psychiatric Research?," *Molecular Psychiatry*, 2011; 16(3): 252–264.

Miller, AH, and CL Raison, "The Role of Inflammation in Depression: From Evolutionary Imperative to Modern Treatment Target," *Nat Rev Immunol*, 2016; 16(1): 22–34.

Perna, G, et al., "Are Anxiety Disorders Associated with Accelerated Aging? A Focus on Neuroprogression," *Neural Plasticity*, 2016; 2016: 8457612.

Poulton, R, et al., "The Dunedin Multidisciplinary Health and Development Study: Overview of the First 40 Years, with an Eye to the Future," *Soc Psychiatry Psychiatr Epidemiol*, 2015; 50(5): 679–693.

Raison, CL, et al., "Neuropsychiatric Adverse Effects of Interferon-Alpha: Recognition and Management," *CNS Drugs*, 2005; 19(2): 105–123.

Salinas, J, et al., "Association of Loneliness with 10-Year Dementia Risk and Early Markers of Vulnerability for Neurocognitive Decline," *Neurology*, 2022.

Sapolsky, RM, LC Krey, and BS McEwen, "Prolonged Glucocorticoid Exposure Reduces Hippocampal Neuron Number: Implications for Aging," *J Neurosci*, 1985; 5(5): 1222–1227.

Vogel, S, and L Schwabe, "Learning and Memory under Stress: Implications for the Classroom," *NPJ Science of Learning*, 2016; 1(1): 16011.

Question 10: Is there medication to treat dementia?

Abner, EL, et al., "Mild Cognitive Impairment: Statistical Models of Transition Using Longitudinal Clinical Data," *Int J Alzheimers Dis,* 2012; 2012: 291920.

Accelerated Approval Program, Accessed July 16, 2021, www.fda.gov/drugs/information-health-care-professionals-drugs/accelerated-approval-program.

Bagley, N, and R Sachs, "The Drug That Could Break American Health Care," *The Atlantic,* 2021.

Bell, J, "Major Health Centers, Insurers Push Back Against Aduhelm Biopharma Dive," 2021.

Birks, J, "Cholinesterase Inhibitors for Alzheimer's Disease," *Cochrane Database Syst* 2006; Rev(1): Cd005593.

Budd Haeberlein, S, et al., "EMERGE and ENGAGE Topline Results: Two Phase 3 Studies to Evaluate Aducanumab in Patients with Early Alzheimer's Disease," *Biogen Investor Report,* 2020.

"Phases of Clinical Trials," 2015, www.australianclinicaltrials.gov.au/what-clinical-trial/phases-clinical-trials.

Cohrs, R, "Medicare Finalizes Its Restrictions on New Alzheimer's Drug, Despite Pressure from Drugmakers," *STAT,* 2022.

Cummings, J, et al., "Alzheimer's Disease Drug Development Pipeline: 2022," *Alzheimer's & Dementia: Translational Research & Clinical Interventions,* 2022; 8(1): e12295.

Dunn, B, P Stein, and P Cavazzoni, "Approval of Aducanumab for Alzheimer Disease: The FDA's Perspective," *JAMA Internal Medicine,* 2021.

Eisai, "Lecanemab Confirmatory Phase 3 Clarity Ad Study Met Primary Endpoint, Showing Highly Statistically Significant Reduction of Clinical Decline in Large Global Clinical Study of 1,795 Participants with Early Alzheimer's Disease," 2022.

Feuerstein, A, and D Garde, "Biogen's Reckoning: How the Aduhelm Debacle Pushed a Troubled Company and Its Fractured Leadership to the Brink," *STAT,* 2021.

Feuerstein, A, M Herper, and D Garde, "Inside 'Project Onyx': How Biogen Used an FDA Back Channel to Win Approval of Its Polarizing Alzheimer's Drug," *STAT+*, 2021.

Feuerstein, AGD, "Biogen to Replace CEO as It 'Substantially' Curbs Spending on Its Alzheimer's Drug," *STAT*, 2022.

Gorenstein, D, "The Aducanumab Aftermath: The Patient Perspective," Tradeoffs.org, June 23, 2021.

Harrison, SL, et al., "The Dispensing of Psychotropic Medicines to Older People Before and After They Enter Residential Aged Care," *Medical Journal of Australia*, 2020; 212(7): 309–313.

Kepplinger, EE, "FDA's Expedited Approval Mechanisms for New Drug Products," *Biotechnol Law Rep*, 2015; 34(1): 15–37.

Kesselheim, A, and J Avorn, "The FDA Has Reached a New Low," *New York Times*, 2021.

Lovelace Jnr, B, "Biogen Stock Falls After FDA Calls for Federal Investigation into Alzheimer's Drug Approval," *CNBC*, July 9, 2021.

"Merformin in Alzheimer's Dementia Prevention (MAP)," www. clinicaltrials .gov/ct2/show/NCT04098666?term=metformin&cond =Dementia&draw=2&rank=2

Raina, P, et al., "Effectiveness of Cholinesterase Inhibitors and Memantine for Treating Dementia: Evidence Review for a Clinical Practice Guideline," *Ann Intern Med*, 2008; 148(5): 379–397.

"Representativeness of Participants Eligible to Be Enrolled in Clinical Trials of Aducanumab for Alzheimer Disease Compared with Medicare Beneficiaries with Alzheimer Disease and Mild Cognitive Impairment," *JAMA*.

Schneider, L, "A Resurrection of Aducanumab for Alzheimer's Disease," *The Lancet Neurology*, 2020; 19(2): 111–112.

Scott IA. "Monoclonal Antibodies for Treating Early Alzheimer Disease—A Commentary on Recent 'Positive' Trials," *Age and Aging.* 2024;53(2).

Sims JR, Zimmer JA, Evans CD, et al. "Donanemab in Early Symptomatic Alzheimer Disease: The TRAILBLAZER-ALZ 2 Randomized Clinical Trial," *JAMA*. 2023;330(6):512-527.

Snyder Bulik, B, "Celeb-Backed Alzheimer's Association Campaign Aims to Build Grassroots Support for Biogen's Aducanumab Ahead of FDA Decision," 2021.

van Dyck CH, Swanson CJ, Aisen P, et al. "Lecanemab in Early Alzheimer's Disease," *N Engl J Med*. 2023;388(1):9-21.

Question 11: What is life like for a person living with dementia?

"Aged Care Workforce Census Report," Department of Health, Australian Government, 2020.

Baber, W, et al., "The Experience of Apathy in Dementia: A Qualitative Study," *Int J Environ Res Public Health*, 2021; 18(6): 3325.

Brodaty, H, BM Draper, and LF Low, "Behavioural and Psychological Symptoms of Dementia: A Seven-Tiered Model of Service Delivery," *Medical Journal of Australia*, 2003; 178(5): 231–234.

"Care Support Guide: Understanding Apathy in People with Dementia," Dementia Support Australia, https://www.dementia.com.au/resource-hub/understanding-apathy-in-people-with-dimentia.

"Interim Report: Neglect, Royal Commission into Aged Care Quality and Safety," Commonwealth of Australia, 2019.

Cuijpers, P, "Depressive Disorders in Caregivers of Dementia Patients: A Systematic Review," *Aging & Mental Health*, 2005; 9(4): 325–330.

Davey, M, "St Basil's Aged Care Inquest Hears Testing Delays After First Covid-19 Case a 'Root Cause' of 50 Deaths," *The Guardian*, 2021.

Finnamore, S, "Dementia Is a Place Where My Mother Lives; It Is Not Who She Is," *New York Times*, 2022.

Informal Carers, September 2021, www.aihw.gov.au/reports/australias-welfare/informal-carers.

Kaspiew, R, R Carson, and H Rhoades, "Elder Abuse: Understanding Issues, Frameworks and Responses," *Australian Institute of Family Studies.*

"Patient Capacity to Consent," Office of the Public Advocate.

Schulz, R, and LM Martire, "Family Caregiving of Persons with Dementia: Prevalence, Health Effects and Support Strategies," *American Journal of Geriatric Psychiatry*, 2004; 12(3): 240–249.

Shaw, SR, et al., "Uncovering the Prevalence and Neural Substrates of Anhedonia in Frontotemporal Dementia," *Brain* 2021; 144(5): 1551–1564.

"Who Cares?," *Four Corners*, ABC, 2018.

Question 12: How should I care for someone with dementia?

https://www.alz.org/media/Documents/alzheimers-facts-and-figures-special-report.pdf

Question 14: Should people with dementia be able to choose end-of-life options for their future selves?

"American Geriatrics Society Feeding Tubes in Advanced Dementia Position Statement," *J Am Geriatr Soc*, 2014; 62(8): 1590–1593.

Asscher, ECA, and S van de Vathorst, "First Prosecution of a Dutch Doctor Since the Euthanasia Act of 2002: What Does the Verdict Mean?," *Journal of Medical Ethics*, 2020; 46(2): 71.

Bomford, A, "Wanting to Die at "Five to Midnight": Before Dementia Takes Over," Accessed 30 March, 2020, www.bbc.com/news/stories-47047579.

Dworkin, R, "Autonomy and the Demented Self," *The Millbank Quarterly*, 1986; 64: 4–16.

Question 15: Can improving diet help avoid dementia?

Akbaraly, T, et al., "Association of Long-Term Diet Quality with Hippocampal Volume: Longitudinal Cohort Study," *American Journal of Medicine*, 2018; 131(11): 1372–1381.

Burckhardt, M, et al., "Souvenaid for Alzheimer's Disease," 2020(12).

Burton, R, and N Sheron, "No Level of Alcohol Consumption Improves Health," *The Lancet*, 2018; 392(10152): 987–988.

Fairfield, KM, et al., "Vitamin Intake and Disease Prevention," 2022.

Hosking, DE, et al,. "MIND Not Mediterranean Diet Related to 12-Year Incidence of Cognitive Impairment in an Australian Longitudinal Cohort Study," *Alzheimer's & Dementia*, 2019; 15(4): 581–589.

Jacka, FN, et al., "A Randomised Controlled Trial of Dietary Improvement for Adults with Major Depression (the 'SMILES' Trial)'," *BMC Medicine*, 2017; 15(1): 23.

Ma, Y, et al., "Higher Risk of Dementia in English Older Individuals Who Are Overweight or Obese," *Int J Epidemiol*, 2020; 49(4): 1353–1365.

Manson, JE, et al., "Marine n–3 Fatty Acids and Prevention of Cardiovascular Disease and Cancer," *New England Journal of Medicine*, 2018; 380(1): 23–32.

Srour, B, et al., "Ultra-Processed Food Intake and Risk of Cardiovascular Disease: Prospective Cohort Study (NutriNet-Santé)," *BMJ*, 2019; 365: l1451.

Stevenson, RJ, et al., "Hippocampal-Dependent Appetitive Control Is Impaired by Experimental Exposure to a Western-Style Diet," *Royal Society Open Science*, 2020; 7(2): 191338.

Valls-Pedret, C, et al., "Mediterranean Diet and Age-Related Cognitive Decline: A Randomized Clinical Trial," *JAMA Internal Medicine*, 2015; 175(7): 1094–1103.

Question 16: Can exercise help to avoid dementia?

Australian Institute of Health and Welfare, *Insufficient Physical Activity*, 2020.

Gleeson, M, et al., "The Anti-Inflammatory Effects of Exercise: Mechanisms and Implications for the Prevention and Treatment of Disease," *Nature Reviews Immunology*, 2011; 11(9): 607–615.

Madore, C, et al., "Microglia, Lifestyle Stress and Neurodegeneration," *Immunity*, 2020; 52(2): 222–240.

Mandolesi, L, et al., "Effects of Physical Exercise on Cognitive Functioning and Wellbeing: Biological and Psychological Benefits," *Frontiers in Psychology*, 2018; 9: 509.

Pentikäinen, H, et al., "Muscle Strength and Cognition in Ageing Men and Women: The DR's EXTRA Study," *European Geriatric Medicine*, 2017; 8(3): 275–277.

"Physical Inactivity," *Global Health Observatory*, Accessed March 5, 2022.

Samieri, C, et al., "Association of Cardiovascular Health Level in Older Age with Cognitive Decline and Incident Dementia," *JAMA*, 2018; 320(7): 657–664.

Sui, SX, et al., "Skeletal Muscle Health and Cognitive Function: A Narrative Review," *Int J Mol Sci*, 2020; 22(1): 255.

Yoon, M, et al., "Association of Physical Activity Level with Risk of Dementia in a Nationwide Cohort in Korea," *JAMA Network Open*, 2021; 4(12): e2138526.

Question 17: Why are challenge and rest so good for our brains?
Gu, F, et al., "Total and Cause-Specific Mortality of US Nurses Working Rotating Night Shifts," *American Journal of Preventive Medicine*, 2015; 48(3): 241–252.

Kirsch, D, "Stages and Architecture of Normal Sleep," February 2022.

Owen, AM, et al., "Putting Brain Training to the Test," *Nature*, 2010; 465: 775.

Sabia, S, et al., "Association of Sleep Duration in Middle and Old Age with Incidence of Dementia," *Nature Communications*, 2021; 12(1): 2289.

Salinas, J, et al., "Association of Loneliness with 10-Year Dementia Risk and Early Markers of Vulnerability for Neurocognitive Decline," *Neurology*, 2022.

Scarmeas, N, et al., "Influence of Leisure Activity on the Incidence of Alzheimer's Disease," *Neurology*, 2001; 57(12): 2236–2242.

Straif, K, et al., "Carcinogenicity of Shift-Work, Painting, and Fire-Fighting," *The Lancet Oncology*, 2007; 8(12): 1065–1066.

Willis, SL, et al., "Long-Term Effects of Cognitive Training on Everyday Functional Outcomes in Older Adults," *JAMA*, 2006; 296(23): 2805–2814.

Zhong, G, et al., "Sleep–Wake Disturbances in Common Neurodegenerative Diseases: A Closer Look at Selected Aspects of the Neural Circuitry," *J Neurol Sci*, 2011; 307(1–2): 9–14.

Question 18: How can your doctor help you prevent dementia?

Anstey, KJ, et al., "Smoking as a Risk Factor for Dementia and Cognitive Decline: A Meta-Analysis of Prospective Studies," *American Journal of Epidemiology*, 2007; 166(4): 367–378.

Australian Institute of Health and Welfare, "Tobacco Smoking," Accessed March 1, 2022.

Cataldo, JK, JJ Prochaska, and SA Glantz, "Cigarette Smoking Is a Risk Factor for Alzheimer's Disease: An Analysis Controlling for Tobacco Industry Affiliation," *J Alzheimers Dis*, 2010; 19(2): 465–480.

"Classification and Diagnosis of Diabetes: Standards of Medical Care in Diabetes: 2021," *Diabetes Care*, 2021; 44(Suppl 1): s15–33.

Laurent, S, and P Boutouyrie, "The Structural Factor of Hypertension," *Circulation Research*, 2015; 116(6): 1007–1021.

Leng, Y, et al., "Association of Sleep-Disordered Breathing with Cognitive Function and Risk of Cognitive Impairment: A Systematic Review and Meta-Analysis," *JAMA Neurol*, 2017; 74(10): 1237–1245.

Li, W, et al., "Type-2 Diabetes Mellitus Is Associated with Brain Atrophy and Hypometabolism in the ADNI Cohort," *Neurology*, 2016; 87(6): 595–600.

Mantzoros, CSS, "Insulin Action," January 2022.

Mueller, NT, et al., "Association of Age with Blood Pressure Across the Lifespan in Isolated Yanomami and Yekwana Villages," *JAMA Cardiology*, 2018; 3(12): 1247–1249.

Question 19: Are poverty and discrimination risk factors for dementia?
"About NACCHO," www.naccho.org.au/about-us.

Adair, T, and AD Lopez, "An Egalitarian Society? Widening Inequalities in Premature Mortality from Non-Communicable Diseases in Australia, 2006–16," *Int J Epidemiol*, 2021; 50(3): 783–796.

Australian Institute of Aboriginal and Torres Strait Islander Studies, *The Stolen Generations*.

Australian Institute of Health and Welfare, "Mortality and Life Expectancy of Indigenous Australians: 2008–2012," AIHW, 2014; Cat no IHW 140.

Cave, L, et al., "Racial Discrimination and Allostatic Load Among First Nations Australians: A Nationally Representative Cross-Sectional Study," *BMC Public Health*, 2020; 20(1): 1881.

Cobb-Clark, DA, "Intergenerational Transmission of Disadvantage in Australia," *Australian Institute of Health and Welfare*, 2019.

Dabelea, D, "The Predisposition to Obesity and Diabetes in Offspring of Diabetic Mothers," *Diabetes Care*, 2007; 30 Suppl 2: S169–174.

Dalfrà, MG, et al., "Genetics and Epigenetics: New Insight on Gestational Diabetes Mellitus," *Frontiers in Endocrinology*, 2020; 11(936).

Eberly, LA, et al., "Identification of Racial Inequities in Access to Specialized Inpatient Heart Failure Care at an Academic Medical Center," *Circulation: Heart Failure*, 2019; 12(11): e006214.

Elliott, ML, et al., "Brain-Age in Midlife is Associated with Accelerated Biological Aging and Cognitive Decline in a Longitudinal Birth Cohort," *Molecular Psychiatry*, 2019.

Harman, K, "Explainer: The Evidence for the Tasmanian Genocide," *The Conversation*, January 18, 2018.

Julia, C, and AJ Valleron, "Louis-René Villermé (1782–1863), a Pioneer in Social Epidemiology: Re-Analysis of His Data on Comparative Mortality in Paris in the Early 19th Century," *Journal of Epidemiology and Community Health*, 2011(1979–); 65(8): 666–670.

Kivimäki, M, et al., "Association Between Socioeconomic Status and the Development of Mental and Physical Health Conditions in Adulthood: A Multi-Cohort Study," *The Lancet Public Health*, 2020; 5(3): e140–e149.

Koye, D, et al, "Guideline-Based Cardiovascular Disease Risk Assessment Among Indigenous Australians in a General Practice Setting," *Int J Epidemiol*, 2021; 50(Supplement 1).

"Lamarckism," *Encyclopedia Britannica*, Accessed September 29, 2021, www.britannica.com/science/Lamarckism.

Logan, JAR, et al., "When Children Are Not Read to at Home: The Million Word Gap," *J Dev Behav Pediatr*, 2019; 40(5): 383–386.

McGowan, M, and C Knaus, "NSW Police Pursue 80% of Indigenous People Caught with Cannabis Through Courts," *The Guardian*, June 10, 2020.

Noble, KG, et al., "Family Income, Parental Education and Brain Structure in Children and Adolescents," *Nat Neurosci*, 2015; 18(5): 773–778.

Pham, TM, et al,. "Trends in Dementia Diagnosis Rates in UK Ethnic Groups: Analysis of UK Primary Care Data," *Clin Epidemiol*, 2018; 10: 949–960.

Poulton, R, et al,. "Association Between Children's Experience of Socioeconomic Disadvantage and Adult Health: A Life-Course Study," *The Lancet*, 2002; 360(9346): 1640–1645.

Radford, K, et al., "Comparison of Three Cognitive Screening Tools in Older Urban and Regional Aboriginal Australians," *Dementia and Geriatric Cognitive Disorders*, 2015; 40(1–2): 22–32.

Ryan L, et al., *Colonial Frontier Massacres in Australia, 1788–1930*, University of Newcastle, 2017–2022.

Sharp, ES, and M Gatz, "Relationship Between Education and Dementia: An Updated Systematic Review," *Alzheimer Disease and Associated Disorders*, 2011; 25(4): 289–304.

Staff, RT, MJ Hogan, and LJ Whalley, "The Influence of Childhood Intelligence, Social Class, Education and Social Mobility on Memory and Memory Decline in Late Life," *Age and Ageing*, 2018; 47(6): 847–852.

Stern, Y, et al., "Rate of Memory Decline in AD Is Related to Education and Occupation: Cognitive Reserve?," *Neurology*, 1999; 53(9): 1942–1947.

Tavella, R, et al., "Disparities in Acute In-hospital Cardiovascular Care for Aboriginal and Non-Aboriginal South Australians," *Medical Journal of Australia*, 2016; 205(5): 222–227.

Trauer, JM, et al., "Understanding How Victoria, Australia Gained Control of Its Second COVID-19 Wave," *Nat Commun*, 2021; 12(1): 6266.

Watts, TW, GJ Duncan, and H Quan, "Revisiting the Marshmallow Test: A Conceptual Replication Investigating Links Between Early Delay of Gratification and Later Outcomes," *Psychological Science*, 2018; 29(7): 1159–1177.

Question 20: How do you avoid the stigma of living with dementia?

Alzheimer's Australia, "Dementia and the Impact of Stigma," 2017.

Andrews, A, P Tucker, and K Waddington, *The History of Bethlem*, New York, Taylor & Francis, 1997.

Dow, A, and L Mannix, "'Shouting and Kicking': Hospitals Reveal New Source of COVID Spread," *The Age*, September 11, 2020.

Evans, SC, "Ageism and Dementia," in L Ayalon and C Tesch-Römer (eds), *Contemporary Perspectives on Ageism*, Springer International Publishing, 2018: 263–275.

Gregorevic, K, et al., "Presenting Symptoms of COVID-19 and Clinical Outcomes in Hospitalised Older Adults," *Intern Med J*, 2021.

Hugo, C, et al., "What Does It Cost to Feed Aged Care Residents in Australia?," *Nutrition & Dietetics*, 2018; 75(1): 6–10.

Kevern, P, "Why Are We So Afraid of Dementia?," *The Conversation*, September 12, 2017.

Killaspy, H, "From the Asylum to Community Care: Learning from Experience," *British Medical Bulletin*, 2007; 79–80(1): 245–258.

Tang, W, et al., "Concern About Developing Alzheimer's Disease or Dementia and Intention to Be Screened: An Analysis of National Survey Data," *Archives of Gerontology and Geriatrics*, 2017; 71: 43–49.

Ward, J, "All in the Family: Tax and Financial Practices of Australia's Largest Family Owned Aged Care Companies," A Tax Justice Network—Australia and Centre for International Corporate Tax Accountability & Research (CICTAR) Report, May 2019.

Conclusion: How do we live well with dementia?

Alzheimer's Society, "The Impact of COVID-19 on People Affected by Dementia," 2020.

"Cognitive Stimulation Theraphy: Enhancing Brain Health," November 15, 2023, cstdementia.com/page/guiding-principles.

"Provisional Mortality Statistics, Provisional Deaths Data for Measuring Changes in Patterns of Mortality During the COVID-19 Pandemic and Recovery Period," Accessed September 9, 2021, www.abs.gov.au /statistics/health/causes-death/provisional-mortality-statistics /latest-release#measuring-excess-deaths.

Suárez-González, A, et al., "The Effect of COVID-19 Isolation Measures on the Cognition and Mental Health of People Living with Dementia: A Rapid Systematic Review of One Year of Quantitative Evidence," *EClinicalMedicine*, 2021; 39.

About the Author

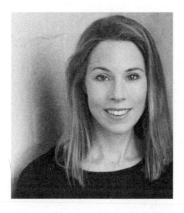

Dr. Kate Gregorevic is a geriatrician and the author of *Staying Alive: The Science of Living Happier, Healthier and Longer*. She has clinical experience looking after people with all stages of dementia and is endlessly fascinated by the ways that physical health intersects with social and emotional health. Kate has also completed a PhD examining the impact of positive psychosocial factors on physical frailty in older adults. Kate lives in Melbourne with her husband and three children.